Advance Appreciation for
Sharing The Care

"Lyn and Bill Roche have done it again! They've come up with a caregiver companion piece that is an easy to understand common sense approach to caring for a loved one. *Sharing The Care* provides simple, positive activities and suggestions that benefit residents, facility personnel and family members alike. The cross-reference topic index is a valuable resource for anyone who is sharing the care. Almost all family caregivers need help with the residual guilt they feel. This book will be very helpful in reducing caregiver guilt and stress because it emphasizes quality visits and ways to stay involved."

—SANDY GEHRMANN, Director, St. Croix County Department on Aging, Hudson, Wisconsin

"Reading *Sharing The Care* is like having a wise friend who provides a great source of practical guidance and courage. It is the perfect gift for supporting a caregiver–family or professional. It's also a must for any friend of a nursing home resident. *Sharing The Care* is packed with excellent tips and ideas. It should be given to every family with a loved one in a care facility."

—BILL GOODRICH, Co-author of *Nursing Home Ministry,* President and Founder, God Cares Ministry, Avon Lake, Ohio

"Some family caregivers say, 'No one else can care for my family as well as me, so these nursing homes had better be really good for the money they charge!' In *Sharing The Care,* Bill and Lyn Roche provide a guide to a different way of thinking and feeling about the role of the nursing home and the caring family. They offer sage advice for establishing the conditions for a team approach to loving care, with the family and the facility staff working together. This is a much needed, thoughtful and loving approach to long term care for a member of your family."

—ROBERT J. DOYLE, Former Executive Director, Southwest Florida Chapter of the Alzheimer's Association, Sarasota, Florida

"The old adage 'less is more' is definitely the case when it comes to *Sharing The Care.* This pocket-sized book is packed with wisdom and encouragement that could only come from someone who has already walked the path that caregivers are facing. It offers daily guidance and inspiration to help caregivers make the transition into being partners with care facilities. Anyone who is a caregiver or looking at that prospect in the future, will appreciate *Sharing The Care.* This insightful book, filled with short bursts of experience, will help all caregivers. While each daily reading takes less than a minute, the lessons they teach will last for a lifetime."

—CARMEN LEAL, Author of *The Twenty-Third Psalm for Caregivers, Faces of Huntington's, and Portraits of Huntington's,* Partner in care with a nursing home, Naples, Florida

"Dad has been in an assisted living facility for one year and though the staff is wonderful, there are still questions and feelings I was at a loss to understand. I have searched for help and *Sharing The Care* with its loving insights and practical suggestions is truly an answer to prayer."

—CAROL HOPKINS, Family Caregiver, Pultneyville, New York

"At last—a resource specifically designed for caregivers who must share the care of their loved ones! In *Sharing The Care,* Lyn and Bill Roche provide words of wisdom and strength for all of us. Placement of someone in a care facility requires special nurturing to all involved. Caregivers will find this book manna for their spirits. Educational and uplifting, these small lessons of love will become a training manual for all who read it, and a sustaining place for caregivers to turn each day."

—VICTORIA McCARTY, Caregiving Specialist, Author and Publisher of Care Tender, a monthly newsletter for caregivers, Camano Island, Washington

"As a nurse and the director of an assisted living facility, I know what a struggle it is for families to reach the decision to place a loved one with us. I believe *Sharing The Care* is a great resource for caregivers. It's a wonderful book!"

—DONNA POWELL, Executive Director, Crown Pointe Assisted Living Community, Sebring, Florida

"As with *Coping With Caring,* Lyn and Bill have once again through *Sharing The Care,* revealed caregiving from a caregiver's perspective. I strongly recommend both books as required resources for all who have the responsibility of care for a loved one. The authors are able to answer the tough questions because as caregivers themselves they have asked them. As the Chaplain of one of the largest multi-level care communities in our area, I am often asked by caregivers for specific resources that will give them hope. Lyn and Bill are my authors of choice. Their love of the Lord and their compassion for caregivers shines through every book, tape and seminar."

—STEVE NYHAN, Chaplain, The Palms of Sebring, Sebring, Florida

"*Sharing The Care* will stimulate your mind to the many facets of caring for an elderly loved one. It targets the simplistic and yet vital steps you can take to make the experience rewarding and productive. The time spent by you and others can help discover a healthy approach to the adult care lifestyle."

—DAVID and WANDA ROBINSON, Senior Pastors, Church of God, Montcalm, West Virginia

"There are plenty of books and booklets designed to help in the selection of a care facility, but *Sharing The Care* is the first we've found to sustain and guide us as we meet the real challenges and changes in our continued role as caregivers for Mom. The insights the authors have from their own personal experiences are valuable beyond measure! Through *Sharing The Care,* we feel someone truly understands and is willing to walk beside us on this part of the journey."

—SHARON and HORACE JAMES, Family Caregivers, Mesa, Arizona

"*Sharing The Care* is an inspirational and exemplary work written with a compassion and wisdom that transcends the mundane and builds caring concepts into all of us! Bill and Lyn Roche have delivered an authentic treasure filled with wisdom born out of life experience that will bless every reader. Their gentle and loving insights are extremely helpful not only for caregivers, but for anyone who faces the challenge of daily ministering to others. Their sensitivity is truly engaging and makes the reader feel that he or she is not alone, that there is someone who has personally faced, and accurately understands caregiving. We found their writing style to be very practical and down to earth, clear and easy to understand, yet, demonstrating an exceptional sensitivity that is truly engaging. *Sharing The Care* speaks to the potential in all of us to become loving, compassionate, knowledgeable, and faithful caregivers!"

—ARLAN and MARY SAPP, Pastors, Restoration Center, Sebring, Florida

"As a 24/7 caregiver for my wife Carol, who has late stage Alzheimer's Disease, I can attest to the value of having such a resource to help the caregiver get through the many trials and tribulations one encounters while providing care for a loved one. Many of the problems encountered in the adult care facility are identical to those in the loved one's home environment. Many of the suggested remedies in *Sharing The Care* can be applied in the home environment as well. From my perspective as a homebound caregiver, I heartily endorse this landmark reference resource for caregivers—whether the loved one is at home or in an adult care facility. All caregivers regardless of the loved one's diagnosis, will benefit from reading this book. It is indeed a 'must read' for all caregivers!"

"As not only a Geriatrician, but as a son to a mother who was a sufferer of Alzheimer's, I find *Sharing The Care* by Lyn and Bill Roche to be extremely insightful, helpful, and inspirational. A family never knows if they are doing the right thing for their loved one when they are placing them in an extended care facility. There is always much soul searching and fear associated with the decision. *Sharing The Care* helps with the transition from one-to-one caregiving, to caregiving as a shared responsibility. I had to make this decision for my mother. My wife Shirley and I cared for her at home for many years. Then when Mother suffered a stroke, the medical doctor in me told me it was time for an extended care facility, but the son in me had many doubts. It would have given me more comfort if I'd had a resource as great as *Sharing The Care.* I plan to use this book for my many patients who are having a hard time reaching a decision about what is best for their loved one. I highly and strongly endorse *Sharing The Care.*"

"Bill and Lyn Roche have written a warm-hearted, insightful, and useful book for all those who care about and for the aging and elderly. It was obviously birthed through their own personal involvement, and so the thoughts come to us already field-tested through years of experience. It is chocked full of practical insights and pointers for loving action. It is organized in easy to read portions, with a valuable index. This book will take much of the unnecessary anxiety and uncertainty out of such caregiving and further enrich anyone's ongoing commitments. It is a companion to keep close at hand through good times and bad. I highly recommend this book for both veterans and newcomers to the growing cadre of caregivers blessed to spend time with the aging elderly."

  —TOM McCORMICK, Co-author *Nursing Home Ministry*, Seminary Professor with over thirty years experience working in nursing homes, Toronto, Ontario, Canada

SHARING THE CARE

When Someone You Love Resides
In An Adult Care Facility

by

LYN and BILL ROCHE

JOURNEY PUBLICATIONS
Avon Park, Florida

Copyright © 2004 By Journey Publications

Scripture taken from the HOLY BIBLE, NEW INTERNATIONAL VERSION®. Copyright© 1973, 1978, 1984 by International Bible Society. Used by permission of Zondervan Publishing House. All rights reserved.

Library of Congress Cataloging in Publication Data
Main Entry Under Title:
Sharing The Care: When Someone You Love Resides In An Adult Care Facility
Roche, Lyn and Bill
1. Caregiving 2. Adult Care Facility 3. Aging
4. Elder Care

LCCN 2004093181
ISBN 0-9754698-0-0

Printed in the United States of America

Cover Design: Journey Publications

In Memory of

Bill, Sr., Ethel,

Gene, Janie,

Gee. . . buttons and bows,

Gam. . . a bushel and a peck. . .

Dedication

This book is lovingly dedicated to
Cheryl and Ralph Gravelle,
for their years of devoted caregiving.

Acknowledgments

Our sincere thanks goes out to all the family members of care facility residents, the many staff members, and the residents who anonymously responded to the questionnaires we circulated while writing *Sharing The Care*. The responses came from all over the United States. Your sharing with us will ultimately help others who either reside in, work in, or have loved ones living in adult long-term care facilities.

We also want to express our appreciation to the many facilities that allowed us to visit often and at all hours.

We lovingly thank all the members of our own family for truly knowing what it is to share the care of loved ones with each other and with caring professionals.

Words printed on this page could never accurately express our heartfelt thankfulness to our Heavenly Father for His guidance and His presence in our lives and work.

Lyn and Bill

Foreword

Sharing The Care deals with aging and the elderly in positive ways. The book casts aging and caring for the elderly in an exciting new light. Years of working together have proven the efforts of compassionate caregivers, be they family members or professionals. We have observed first-hand how care facilities are moving toward the future. Active residents' councils form valuable liaisons between families and care professionals. Forward thinking architectural treatments consider the aesthetics of a home-like environment. The introduction of pets, vegetation, and community as a regular presence vastly improves both residents' and care professionals' emotional and physical well being on a daily basis.

Each facility we visited shared its own unique character. Many made us think, "I would be happy here!" How exciting!

Bill Roche

Introduction

How to Use This Book

Sharing The Care is written from a family member's point of view, but is clearly meant to be read by anyone who works in, lives in, or visits someone in an adult long-term care facility. Long term includes assisted living facilities, nursing homes, and any congregate living setting that is a loved one's permanent dwelling, not intended just for short-term rehabilitation or physical therapy.

You may have been the primary caregiver of a loved one before the move to a care facility. This book deals with the adjustments you and your loved one must make. It stresses the value of establishing a successful partnership with the professional caregivers who now also play an important role in the care of your loved one.

The reflections on the top half of each page come from our personal family experiences and from feelings and concerns other caregivers have shared with us. The lower half of each page presents things to consider which are meant to uplift all aspects of caring for the elderly.

It is our desire to offer on-going daily support to anyone involved in care facilities. In the research of the book we found numerous active resident councils. We hope the residents themselves will find this book edifying and helpful.

Sharing The Care is designed to be used in a number of different ways, depending on personal preference and needs. The contents may be read as daily reflections. Or, they can be read straight through. Utilizing the index section for quick access to help with challenges as they occur, makes *Sharing The Care* an ideal reference book.

Like our first book, *Coping With Caring* ISBN 0-943873-29-0 published by Elder Books in 1996, you may wish to read the book first in its entirety and then use it as a daily reflection book throughout the year. Many readers tell us they continue to use it year after year. Unlike the first edition of

Coping With Caring, Sharing The Care does not date each page. However, if page one is used for January 1ˢᵗ you will find the readings of each page will in many cases reflect the appropriate day of the year. For instance, page 365 will fall on New Year's Eve. We do suggest, however, if your loved one is about to become or has just become a resident of a long term adult care facility, you will want to begin with the first page of the text because the opening pages deal with the unique adjustments associated with the newness of the situation. *Sharing The Care* is dedicated to helping make the transition a smooth one for all parties—family members, their loved ones, and the care facility personnel.

The in-depth reflections and tips in *Sharing The Care* intend to make it a resource book for Pastors, Stephen Ministers, outreach groups of many organizations, local and long-distance friends and relatives of residents, and caregivers of all kinds.

It is our sincere prayer that this book be a blessing to you.

Lyn Roche

[4]Love is patient, love is kind. It does not envy, it does not boast, it is not proud. [5]It is not rude, it is not self-seeking, it is not easily angered, it keeps no record of wrongs. [6]Love does not delight in evil but rejoices with the truth. [7]It always protects, always trusts, always hopes, always perseveres.

[8]Love never fails.

—1 CORINTHIANS 13:4-8

Sharing the Care

So many changes—changes in my loved one, changes in me, and now, changes in my role as caregiver. I have to view things from a different perspective. I'm overseeing my loved one's care. I'm sharing the care with caring professionals. We must all work together to help make the merger a smooth one. I'm part of a team now!

Consider this: It's important your relative be involved in as much of the move to the care facility as possible. Don't do everything for her. Let her decide what personal belongings, furnishings, and decorations are to go in her room. She may wish to put something on her door that personalizes it and helps her identify it easily. If she has dementia, you might have to make most of the decisions, but give her as many choices as you can without confusing her.

Sharing the Care

I've left five-year-olds at kindergarten, eleven-year-olds at summer camp, and eighteen-year-olds at college. None of those experiences come close to the first day I left my loved one at the care facility. I felt awful! Perhaps I attached too much finality to it.

Consider this: Unfortunately, our society has viewed long-term care facility placement as an ending. We are learning it can bring many fresh beginnings. New friendships often form between residents. New and better family relationships can emerge when professionals are performing the chores of daily caregiving. Our attitudes and expectations can greatly influence our loved ones' views of the care facility experience.

Sharing the Care

Newness requires patience and understanding on the part of everyone. My loved one is adjusting to a new home. It's a big adjustment for me, too. There are lots of new things for both of us.

Consider this: Realize your relative has new people, surroundings, and schedules to relate to. He may feel overwhelmed. He could be tired from the move and the change. You know him best. He might need you with him quite a bit in the early days. Or, he may need time without you to get acquainted on his own. Be careful not to monopolize his time, but don't let him feel abandoned either. Balance is important for both of you.

Sharing the Care

My loved one is a very important part of our family. The special way we treat her and the loving concern we show her help the staff and her new friends see her for the individual she is.

Consider this: The care facility staff will come to know and respect your relative, hopefully as you do. You may be able to help them get to know her better by sharing some of the important aspects of her life. There are many ways you can choose to do this. You might want to hang a picture history of her on the wall of her room or provide her with a personalized photo album to share.

Sharing the Care

Everyone needs a support system. The number of years lived does not seem to change or negate this basic need. I try to be sensitive and respond to the level of support my loved one needs. I listen and let her know I care.

Consider this: Depending on what is going on in our lives, we seem to require different levels of support from those close to us. In the adjustment period of moving into a care facility, your loved one may require a great deal of attention and reassurance from family and friends. As the new surroundings become more familiar, your relative's normal sense of independence and comfort level will most likely return to normal.

Sharing the Care

I'm doing everything I can to accept my loved one's new home. It's a big change for both of us. New relationships are being formed. There are staff members and new neighbors for all of us to become acquainted with.

Consider this: Family members can feel closer to the surroundings by making a point of learning the names of residents and greeting them with a smile and perhaps a handshake or a gentle pat on the back, hand, or arm. Somehow when you take the time to look into another human being's eyes and address them by name, other issues fall away. A connection forms.

Sharing the Care

Before my loved one moved into the care facility I was almost worn out worrying about her and caring for her. Now, somehow I feel like I need to be doing more. It's a strange thing, I feel guilty and I don't know why.

Consider this: As caring family members, we must realize we are doing all we can and our best is good enough. If we could make our loved ones young again and completely healthy and happy, we would—but we can't. What we can do, is bring plenty of love and joy to the time we now spend with them. We have a marvelous opportunity to be genuinely attentive to the things we can do for them in this new setting.

Sharing the Care

I try not to let little things disturb me. I choose my battles. The overall quality of care is the important issue. Our family works with the staff toward finding positive solutions to any problems we encounter.

Consider this: Many families choose a family spokesperson—often the person who provided primary care prior to the move to the care facility. Usually the spokesperson is the person named in the loved one's legal health care directive as his proxy or surrogate. The designated person must be easily available for staff to reach in an emergency and be able to attend all the regularly scheduled care planning meetings. This representative should share pertinent information with other interested members of the family. Having one person in this role also makes it easier on the staff and shows consideration of their time.

Sharing the Care

Making new friends has never been easy for my loved one. This was a concern regarding her move to the care facility. Our family cannot be with her all the time and we hope she will be able to form meaningful friendships in her new surroundings.

Consider this: Talk to the staff about your relative's life and interests. Ask them if there are residents with similar backgrounds and interests. Suggest the staff help establish conversations between your relative and other residents. When you visit, try to conveniently place your relative near the residents you feel she may be drawn to socially.

Sharing the Care

My presence is very important to my loved one and to the facility staff. We're all a team and we work well together. My role as a caring member plays a very significant part in my relative's comfort level.

Consider this: You may find there are things the professional caregivers don't do for your loved one due to lack of time and the amount of work they are expected to get done on their shifts. Observation on your part will make you aware of special things you can do for your relative that staff just cannot do. Family and friends should do individual caregiving needs such as the straightening of dresser drawers, mending, quality conversations, and leisurely walks with your loved one.

Sharing the Care

I work a traditional 8:00 to 5:00 job—Monday through Friday. It's difficult for me to get time off during the day. I usually visit my loved one on a Saturday or Sunday afternoon. I mail cheery notes to her when I can during the week.

Consider this: Many facilities realize there are some family members who are unable to attend anything the facility schedules during the week. Occasionally, care-planning meetings can be set up on a Saturday when weekday appointments are impossible for the family primary caregiver. If you are in this situation, talk to the administrator and see if you can arrange meeting times that are mutually convenient.

Sharing the Care

I wish I had more time to spend with my loved one. There doesn't always seem to be adequate time, but the time we do have together is enjoyable.

Consider this: Busy schedules and active lives can make it difficult to include enough time to visit relatives in care facilities as often as we'd like to. Large families often work out a schedule together and no one person feels all the burden. Smaller families can encourage their relative's friends to make regular visits. Families who live a long distance away often contact organizations with active volunteers who befriend long-term care facility residents. Newsy letters from long-distance family members sent on a regular basis can help bridge the miles and retain loving ties.

Sharing the Care

My loved one complains that he cannot converse with the people around him. Many of the residents have handicaps or dementia which prevent them from communicating with him. He is constantly searching for someone to share a mutually satisfying conversation.

Consider this: Daily companionship and comfortable relationships are important to most of us. Changes in residency make it necessary to form new connections. In a care facility, finding new friends can sometimes be difficult. Be sensitive to your relative's needs. Make the staff aware of his desire to be around others with whom he can meaningfully communicate.

Sharing the Care

The cost of long-term care is a burden, but we have no alternative. For the most part, the expenses are understandable. Our family does everything we can to stay within our means and provide our loved one with the best of care.

Consider this: No one likes surprises on a monthly bill. Make sure you know ahead of time if the facility charges for extra services such as helping to feed the residents. Many facilities let family members bring in items like incontinent garments, bed and chair pads, cosmetics, and personal care products. Doing your loved one's laundry yourself in your home usually amounts to a significant savings.

Sharing the Care

I look for what is right, not what is wrong. I have always tried to do this and will continue to do so in this new environment. I realize congregate living is still congregate living no matter how home-like it appears.

Consider this: An apparent lack of privacy can be a concern for your relative and her visitors. Some residents find it difficult to entertain when distracted by activities and noise. The presence of a roommate could even present a problem. Seek out quiet corners in the common areas. When the weather permits, take walks outdoors. Sit in the garden or patio area.

Sharing the Care

I keep wishing my loved one was back home. But even if I close my eyes real hard, the problems won't disappear. Changes have occurred. Things are not like they used to be.

Consider this: Professional caregivers often report that family members experience different degrees of denial. They may not admit their loved one has limitations or a serious illness. The reality of the need for long-term care is often hard to accept. Many diseases such as Alzheimer's disease are progressive and cunning. Acceptance takes time.

Sharing the Care

I encourage my loved one to maintain ties with her community and with other family members. This connection is an important element for maintaining her identity and self-worth.

Consider this: You can be an integral link between your relative and the world outside the care facility. If writing is difficult for her, help her correspond with family members and friends by having her dictate her letters to you. If she no longer speaks but is able to communicate to you by nodding or smiling, try producing short letters for her. Read everything out loud to get her approval before sealing the envelopes and mailing them.

Sharing the Care

In some ways my loved one's new home has become my home, too. I have a strong feeling for the place and spend quality time there. Like his homes of the past, I want to be a part of it and help make it comfortable and secure for him.

Consider this: Many family caregivers volunteer in the care facility. Extra help is usually welcomed. Some family members like to accompany residents and staff on field trips. Others assist with crafts or entertainment. You might want to find out the home's disaster plans. You may be able to join your relative during an emergency and be a big help at a time when the facility needs extra hands.

Sharing the Care

My visits can be reassuring for my loved one and me. They strengthen the bond between us. This living arrangement may not be what either of us wanted or anticipated. Circumstances beyond our control made it necessary for us to seek this level of care. We may both be mourning the loss of a way of life no longer possible. We sit and hold hands and support one another.

Consider this: It's important not to take your relative's negative comments personally. You are doing everything you can for her. Allow her to mourn her losses and let her know her feelings are okay. If you are experiencing excessive guilt feelings, trouble sleeping, or unmanageable stress over the situation, professional or pastoral counseling may be in order to keep yourself healthy. You deserve the best care, too!

Sharing the Care

I don't have unrealistic expectations. This applies to my loved one, the staff, and myself. We are all human. We all deserve the benefit of the doubt and a little slack now and then.

Consider this: The care facility is a real community. It has its strengths and its weaknesses. It consists of staff and residents with their own personal strengths and weaknesses. The facility may be the logical answer or solution for your relative's needs, but that doesn't mean it will be perfect. If you expect it to be perfect, you will be disappointed and cause yourself much anxiety.

Sharing the Care

I cannot make another person happy. I hope my presence and my visits are positive and uplifting for my relative, but they are not his sole existence. He has a life and relationships apart from his relationship with me. He is still responsible for his own attitude and view of life.

Consider this: We are all responsible for our own happiness. This doesn't stop when someone becomes elderly or moves into a care facility. If your relative is confused or has dementia, you can help avoid the things that agitate or upset him. You can be supportive, cheerful, and loving, but you still are not responsible for his happiness. You did not cause his condition. It is not in your control. By maintaining a good attitude and being responsible for your own happiness, you are doing the best you can.

Sharing the Care

My loved one doesn't live in the past, however she enjoys pleasant memories. We often talk about the highlights of her life. She glows and beams in remembrance of them.

Consider this: A large photo of an important event in your relative's life—such as her wedding picture—may be appropriately hung outside the door to her room. Consider placing it in a Plexiglas frame that can be securely screwed into the wall. It will be protected and won't fall or disappear. A picture from the past may help someone with dementia identify their own room more easily.

Sharing the Care

I can't replace my relative's lost friends. I still maintain my place in the family and the relationship I always had with him. But, I can laugh with him and enjoy remembering some of the good times he experienced with his friends in the past.

Consider this: Encourage your relative to make new friends among the other residents. Search for common grounds such as places they've lived, similar work histories, and shared interests to begin conversations and interaction. Often older people worry they have nothing interesting to talk about. Help build up your relative's self-esteem. Keep him informed of things he might find of interest to talk about with his new friends. This will also show your continued interest in him as a social person.

Sharing the Care

The homes I have lived in have not been interior decorators' dreams. I'm happy to say they have been places of comfort filled with well-used furniture and belongings. They've been homes where friends and family congregate and join each other in sharing and caring about one another.

Consider this: A row of occupied chairs or wheelchairs in the hallway or activity center can be more meaningful in terms of sociability than a facility where everything is lovely—but everyone is alone in their own rooms. Lounges with ongoing checker and chess games, jigsaw puzzles, and even spirited discussions among residents are the sign of a healthy, normal home. Comfortable furnishings are more inviting than elaborately decorated community rooms that all look alike!

Sharing the Care

It's extremely necessary my loved one be surrounded by things that were always important to him. He no longer communicates his needs to us. We must rely upon our memories of what meant the most to him throughout his lifetime.

Consider this: If your relative's faith and spiritual convictions were a part of his life, make sure they continue to be. Pray out loud with him, if you have done so together in the past. Provide tapes of his favorite hymns, scriptures, sermons, and teachings. If he is able to attend his church's or synagogue's services, make transportation arrangements for him to do so. Radio and television ministries may be pleasing to him. Be sensitive to his spiritual needs.

Sharing the Care

Part of my job as a family member of a care facility resident is to show support to both my relative and to the staff members. When asked to participate with my relative's care plan, I try to be as honest and objective as possible. I am realistic about his abilities, behavior, and personality. I offer any information and suggestions that I believe will aid in his care and help make the staff's job a little easier.

Consider this: The old saying, "There are two sides to every story," often applies to the care facility situation. If your relative complains about some aspect of his care, listen attentively and reassure him you'll look into it. Check it out objectively before rushing to conclusions. Try to see the whole picture. You'll be better able to help improve the situation and overcome the problem.

Sharing the Care

Personal appearance plays an important part in everyone's self-esteem. When we present a clean, pleasant appearance we feel better all over. Our confidence is boosted!

Consider this: Well-groomed hair, trimmed nails, and clean-shaven faces for the gentlemen never lose their importance. You may wish to take an active role in maintaining your relative's appearance. Visits to the barbershop or beauty salon can be given as gifts. Don't forget sincere compliments go a long way and can help your loved one retain self-esteem and self-interest.

Sharing the Care

The congregate living experience is teaching me a great deal about values in life. I walk through the door and material things lose their importance. My loved one and I are stripped of all the worldly trappings that once surrounded us and affected our relationship in the past.

Consider this: Naturally, your relative wants some of his favorite things around him, but space is limited. Wearing expensive jewelry is no longer wise or practical for him. Giving him expensive gifts is not a good idea, as things can disappear easily. Life in a care facility may be more simplistic than you are both used to, but it can be a real advantage if you realize giving and sharing unconditional love and attention are what is most valued.

Sharing the Care

Some days I just don't feel like visiting. I'm not always cheerful. In fact, sometimes I need some cheering up myself. I have my own problems. I've never been good at pretending and my loved one can see through it if I try to feign a lightness I don't feel.

Consider this: Sometimes you might decide it's just not a good day to visit. Other days you may find a visit with your relative is just what you need. She may still be sensitive to your feelings and your needs, but be careful not to overwhelm her or burden her with your problems. You also need to be good to yourself regarding visits. If you feel obligated, you will develop and harbor resentment. Your visiting schedule should be reasonable and in the proper perspective with the rest of your life and responsibilities.

Sharing the Care

My loved one needs me in new ways. It's not always easy or possible for her to be responsible for details or written records. She may be more confused now, or the lack of space and privacy make it difficult for her to handle all the complexities she did in the past.

Consider this: Naturally you or another family member has taken over certain responsibilities. Some of them such as obtaining a Durable Power of Attorney, Health Care Proxy, and a Living Will were probably worked out prior to the move to the care facility. The family member who accepted those responsibilities should keep copies of all papers pertaining to your relative's care, including forms giving permission for flu shots or pneumonia shots— as well as the facility's monthly bills.

Sharing the Care

Lately my loved one has exhibited some difficult forms of behavior. It's best if I don't overreact. I know there must be some underlying reason for the uncharacteristic, disturbing conduct. I've decided to play detective and try to uncover the real problem.

Consider this: With some effort on your part you will usually be able to discover the cause of difficult behavior, whether your loved one suffers with a form of dementia or not. If the move to the care facility was recent, he may feel unsettled and his fears or frustrations are presenting themselves in an unacceptable manner. Or, it could be a means of getting attention he feels he is not receiving. Work with the staff, spend time with your relative in an attempt to uncover his feelings, and be observant of things that could possibly be upsetting him.

Sharing the Care

Peace and comfort are the things my loved one seems to need the most. We share a spiritual closeness we never experienced before. We've learned to acknowledge reality and be honest with each other. I am privileged to be sharing this special time with her.

Consider this: There are events in life that have great meaning. Although we often refrain from talking about death, the closing period of life is one of the most meaningful. If your relative is terminally ill, acquaint yourself with the philosophy and services of your local Hospice organization. Ask them for a copy of the Bill of Rights for the Dying. Hospice often works closely with care facilities within the facility premises. They also continue to help family members during bereavement.

Sharing the Care

Pleasing surroundings help deepen our inner peace. Most of us strive for such qualities in our homes. My loved one's new home is no exception. I will do all I can to help make her home serene and pleasant.

Consider this: Fresh flowering plants can add a lot to your relative's room and to her mood. A pretty bedspread from home could help give the room a cozy look and also help her identify her own bed more easily. Cassette recordings of favorite music and pleasant posters or wall hangings can be calming and reassuring.

Sharing the Care

When I visit with my loved one, I stress the positives and talk in a positive manner. I find it helps his attitude. Instead of saying, "I miss you," I tell him how much I've looked forward to our visit. There is a difference and the effect it has on him is uplifting, not negative or depressing.

Consider this: A bird feeder outside your relative's window is a loving gift that will continue to bring enjoyment. Consider a small feeder that attaches to the outside window with suction cups. Some are made with a one-way mirror enabling anyone inside to view the birds feeding while the birds see only their own reflections. Keep the feeder filled with seed when you visit and provide a bird book for identifying species.

Sharing the Care

Our family does everything we can to act in our loved one's best interests. Whenever possible we rely on his wishes. Some he still voices. Some he voiced in the past and we abide by them.

Consider this: Obviously, decisions are easier when residents of long-term care facilities have provided specific legal directives regarding their care. Don't be hesitant to talk to the facility administration and your relative's physician about life-sustaining treatments, withdrawal of treatments, do-not-resuscitate orders, and the use of feeding tubes. Clarify what the terms mean to you and to the facility. Make sure you both have a clear understanding. Be familiar with the laws and policies regarding these issues.

Sharing the Care

I try to enrich the present experience. I look for ways to link happy times in the past to happy times now. Today may be different—but not all bad. I don't make comparisons. I just make the best of every day. When I look back at this time I can have happy memories, too.

Consider this: On your next visit, bring tea or special coffee in a thermos and have a party. Help make it a memorable occasion by including pretty cups, linen napkins, and favorite sweets. Ask your relative if she'd like to invite some of her new friends to join in the fun!

Sharing the Care

One essential item needs to be brought with me every time I visit my loved one. The all-important item is my sense of humor. It is often a lifesaver! If I leave it at home, my visit can be a disaster.

Consider this: An easy laugh and a smile make the environment more pleasant for everyone. If your relative seems to have misplaced her sense of humor, perhaps you can help her find it. You may be able to get her to see things from a more cheerful point of view. You might also need your sense of humor to accept her behavior or attitude on any given day.

Sharing the Care

Order has always been an important part of my loved one's life. He is organized and tends to relate to certain routines. Changing a habit is not easy for him.

Consider this: Once your relative's room is set up, it's wise not to rearrange things—especially without his approval and without good reason. Keep things in the same place. Labeling dresser drawers and closets can be a good idea in this new setting, particularly if your relative seems confused or forgetful. When making labels, be sure the letters are big and use a wide dark-colored marker on light-colored paper.

Sharing the Care

I realize I have to let my loved one love me. This isn't a one-way street. She needs to show her love for me. By accepting her affection, I am validating her self-worth. She still has a lot of herself to give—regardless of her environment. I am fortunate to be loved by such a special person and I tell her so!

Consider this: Cotton throws, hand-knit or crocheted lap robes, and shawls are all excellent gifts for people who use wheelchairs. They provide warmth and are short enough not to get caught in the wheels. Keeping laundry day and disappearances in mind, make sure your relative has an ample supply of these items.

Sharing the Care

I don't take my loved one's moods personally. There is a lot more going on in her life besides her relationship with me. So why should I think I am so important to be the cause of her moods? I treat her with love and respect. Her mood is up to her. I do, however, try to uncover what is upsetting her and I work with her and the staff to hopefully improve the situation.

Consider this: The inability to hear well can cause agitation and make someone's behavior or mood appear difficult. Have your relative's hearing checked if you think this could be a problem. Also be aware some of us have selective hearing—we only hear what we choose to hear!

Sharing the Care

My loved one has always had a strong spiritual side. It has not changed with age. In fact, I believe it has become stronger and even more important to her. Recognizing her spiritual connections and needs is vitally important.

Consider this: The care facility probably has a chapel. They may offer religious services, Bible studies, and singing of hymns for the residents throughout the week. Ask your relative if she would enjoy these activities. You might wish to accompany her. If you are unable to join her, keep her informed of the times and meeting places. Let the staff or chaplain know of her desire to attend.

Sharing the Care

I keep my loved one connected with the family. I share up-to-date happenings with him. We enjoy looking at recent photos together. We talk about resemblances and family traits. It helps reaffirm his importance. He will always be a part of us!

Consider this: If your relative spoke a language other than English in his earlier years, he may enjoy speaking or singing songs in that language. If you know of other residents, family members, or staff who speak the language, encourage verbal exchanges with each other. It could be quite comforting and enjoyable. New bonds can be formed.

Sharing the Care

I look at my loved one's folded hands. Hands that were once busy, creative, and loving. They are still loving as she reaches for mine when I arrive and waves good-bye to me when I have to leave. They are the once beautiful hands that still need other hands to hold, activities to do, and pretty things to touch. Sometimes I just hold her hands gently in mine—sometimes I bring them to my face and kiss them.

Consider this: Elderly people who no longer walk can be very active with their hands. Bring photo albums, paper and colored pens for drawing, and cards to play. Consider her level of dexterity and use your imagination! Don't forget ladies love to have their hands manicured and fingernails painted. You may want to provide this service yourself or have it done in the facility's beauty salon.

Sharing the Care

When I visit with my relative I try to be aware of things she may need—physical things as well as emotional needs. I look around her room. I observe how things work or don't work for her. Part of my role is seeing her needs are met and helping her life run smoothly.

Consider this: Some residents have small items they like to carry with them when they leave their rooms. A small bag or basket can be attached to a walker or to the arm of a wheelchair. Canvas bags made especially for wheelchairs and walkers can be purchased through handicap equipment stores or specialty catalogs. One family caregiver knits pouch-shaped bags out of washable rug yarn. She has made them in many different colors to match her relative's clothing. They are more practical than bulky purses.

Sharing the Care

My relationship with my loved one is not the only relationship I have in the care facility. I am building solid relationships with the people I come in contact with there. Other residents, their families, and the staff have greatly enlarged my circle of friends and acquaintances. We are all a part of this special community.

Consider this: If staff members don't wear nametags, suggest they do. Changes in staff and shifts make it difficult to know everyone by name. Be friendly and introduce yourself to staff, residents, and families. Using someone's name facilitates good communication.

Sharing the Care

I still do many things by the trial and error method. I also realize something that worked last week may not work this week. Something that works for someone else's loved one or family may not work for ours. We have individual circumstances—even when we share the same care facility.

Consider this: Some families are successful in taking their loved ones out of the facility for a shopping trip, a restaurant meal, or a visit to a family member's home. Others are not. Outings can prove to be confusing, unrewarding, and exhausting for everyone involved. You will learn what is best in your situation.

Sharing the Care

I hope my loved one's care is good. I hope I am a positive force in his life. There are some things I can't change. I am moving forward with a positive attitude. I have hope in the present—and in the future.

Consider this: Make sure you are doing some fun things for yourself! Just because your relative is unable to do the things you once enjoyed together, does not mean you shouldn't go on enjoying them. If your situations were reversed, wouldn't you want him to continue to participate in the things that bring him pleasure?

Sharing the Care

I have not given up my caregiving responsibilities. I am my loved one's advocate now. I speak on her behalf regarding her needs and wishes. My responsibilities may have changed, but they are just as important and worthy of my best efforts.

Consider this: It's important to stay closely involved with all aspects of your relative's care. Her medical and emotional care still need your attention and will be better because you are overseeing them with love and concern.

Sharing the Care

Caregivers are adjusters. I often have to adjust to my loved one. Sometimes when I visit he is actively participating in an activity. Other times he is quietly observing. There are even times he is hostile to his environment. Not all visits are the same. They are not all enjoyable. I remember not to take things personally.

Consider this: Sometimes, watching an activity can be as fulfilling as participating in it. No one reacts well to being pushed or forced into joining. If an invitation to participate is turned down today, he may choose to be a part of the activity another day. Don't be distressed or surprised if your relative doesn't partake of every activity offered him.

Sharing the Care

There are many advantages to the change in my caregiving role. Before my relative's move to the facility, the physical aspects were becoming exhausting and dangerous for both of us. I could no longer lift him and often when he fell I would fall also. Now his increasing physical needs are met by professionals. I am free from those stresses and can concentrate on other aspects of his care.

Consider this: Many family caregivers find they begin feeling better both emotionally and physically when the physical work of caregiving is taken over by the care facility. It's not unusual for the refreshed caregiver to wonder if she should move her loved one back home and begin daily caregiving again. This is generally not a good idea. It could be a step backward for everyone!

Sharing the Care

I'm aware of changes in the physical aspects of the care facility. I point out changes in furniture arrangement, changes in meeting places, and repair or maintenance work to my loved one. Whenever possible I accompany him to new meeting places or new facilities in the building. I help him identify landmarks and suggest ways to remember the new arrangement.

Consider this: Whatever you can do to help boost and maintain your relative's self-esteem and security will be greatly appreciated. Poor eyesight, confusion, and fear of the unknown can keep him from reaching out and enjoying all the facility has to offer. A few minutes of your time and effort might make a big difference!

Sharing the Care

Light is usually a positive thing. Sunlight, daylight, and soft warm lights are reassuring. They brighten our spirits. Some people just seem to radiate light. They uplift our spirits. I'd like to be a bright ray of light for others!

Consider this: As people age they tend to need more light to see. There should be plenty of natural light in your relative's room and in the care facility as a whole. Bright colors such as yellow and orange are generally easier to see than blue and green. Someone might appear to be confused when the problem is actually due to poor eyesight or inadequate lighting.

Sharing the Care

I try to vary the times of day I visit. This enables me to learn more about the care facility and how it operates. It also makes me aware of my relative's daily routine. I observe how he functions at different times of the day.

Consider this: Some family members make it a habit to just drop in to visit. They often come in unexpected by staff or their loved ones. They feel it gives them more insight and a better picture of what goes on.

Sharing the Care

My loved one tells me she is not happy. This makes me feel guilty and sad, even though I know I can't do anything to make her happy. Is she really unhappy? Or is she pushing my buttons? Am I letting her push my buttons?

Consider this: Ask various staff members how your relative acts when you're not there. You might consider observing her when she doesn't know you're there and is not expecting you. You could very well find her being quite social and acting very happy. If this is the case, try discussing it with her. Tell her how her negative comments make you feel.

Sharing the Care

Exercise is important for all of us. When my loved one and I visit we often walk together. Sometimes we do mild exercises. Our needs may be different, but I enjoy doing activities with him. Besides, every workout I do helps me!

Consider this: Dementia patients may do physical therapy more readily if the activity is associated with something familiar—such as walking from a chair to the bed. A confused person is not likely to follow or remember the directions required for most physical therapy exercises. The everyday therapy of getting up and dressed is very important for patients who have Alzheimer's disease or similar types of dementia.

Sharing the Care

Evenings and nights can be lonely. There is usually less activity going on. Sometimes I look forward to a quiet evening alone to put my feet up and relax. Other times I need to make some plans. I reach out and call someone who may also want company.

Consider this: Find out if the care facility has informal activities for the residents in the evenings. If not, perhaps you could organize some game playing, sing-a-longs, bingo, or movie watching. A regularly scheduled weekly family night might be fun for all. Be sure to check with the staff first. Keep in mind what hour they begin helping the residents get ready for bed.

Sharing the Care

Feeling needed and helpful is a part of feeling good about ourselves. I know my relative needs me in many ways. I let her know that I need her, too. I rely on her wisdom. I need our quiet conversations. Her serenity often rubs off on me.

Consider this: Many able residents still volunteer their time and talents to help others. One lady knits for the Red Cross. Another reads the newspaper to her blind roommate each morning. Residents often take turns raising and bringing in the flag every day. In some facilities they regularly set and clear the tables in the dining room. If your relative has always enjoyed helping others, encourage her to keep on doing so.

Sharing the Care

Demands and stress can cause burn out in anyone. Increased caregiving chores certainly took their toll on me. I am aware of the demands on professional caregivers. They can also get burned out. I will do everything I can to support them and pat them on the back for the great job they do!

Consider this: Most facilities have regularly scheduled in-service classes for their staff. Talk to the in-service director if you have an idea or a need you feel could be addressed at one of their sessions or workshops. If you suggest something that might benefit the residents and staff, they'll most likely consider it and appreciate your interest.

Sharing the Care

I don't burden the staff with our family problems. Every family has some. We are no different. We try to appropriately resolve our problems. When there is something we feel the staff needs to know in order to give our relative the best care possible, our family spokesperson talks with the administrator about it.

Consider this: Old unresolved issues may require professional help. New ways of relating may be learned. If there is someone whose presence upsets or might endanger a resident, the facility needs to be alerted. In extreme situations, legal restraining orders have been used to prohibit certain persons from visiting.

Sharing the Care

Watching seeds sprout and flowers bloom gives hope to the human spirit. Life is represented. The natural order of living is affirmed.

Consider this: If your relative's room has a sunny window, consider planting seeds together. Bring in pots, small gardening tools, and a watering can. The activity may inspire memories and conversations of gardens of the past or life on a farm. Watering and caring for the windowsill garden can prove to be a source of pride and an interest for your relative. Seeing new plant life emerge from the soil can brighten up winter days!

Sharing the Care

Our family tries to space our visits. We realize too many people at one time can overwhelm our loved one. When we all come at one time, we often start talking to each other and he doesn't get the attention he needs. We plan our visits so he will see each of us often, but in small doses.

Consider this: If your relative suffers from dementia, he can become distracted by too many people in the room. Conversations are hard to follow. Identifying individuals will be more difficult for him. Everyone could end up frustrated! One-on-one encounters are more satisfying for someone who is easily upset or confused.

Sharing the Care

Good-byes are difficult. It has always been hard for my loved one and me to leave each other. Now we share little good-byes at the close of every visit. Some days I think it is getting easier. Some days it is hard for both of us.

Consider this: Many family caregivers find it easier to leave when their relative is weary or ready for a nap. A long walk together at the end of the visit could help the resident relax. Saying good-bye from a common area where activities are in progress often works well with dementia patients.

Sharing the Care

Every person, every family, and every situation is unique. I don't compare myself to others. The care I give my loved one and the care she receives from professionals are different in many ways. This doesn't make one better than the other. It is necessary we work together—not against one another.

Consider this: Care facilities differ in the care they offer, the rates they charge, and in their physical appearance. They each possess unique qualities. What appeals to one individual or family may not to another. Be careful not to criticize other facilities.

Sharing the Care

I can help with the quality of my loved one's care by sharing her likes and dislikes with the staff. This might be in the area of foods or activities. When I am able to suggest possible solutions to problems they may be having regarding my loved one, I do so based on things that have worked in the past.

Consider this: Keeping a light on in your relative's room might prevent her from being disoriented if she awakens during the night. Also, playing soft instrumental music through the night can be comforting. Be sure to let the staff know of things your relative is accustomed to—especially the things that reassure her.

Sharing the Care

An aging face is a story, a book—a history all in itself. I study my loved one's face. I explore its history. I see beneath the sagging and the wrinkles to the wealth of experience and understanding within. I ask him questions. I listen. I open the pages while I can!

Consider this: There are a number of reminiscence activities to engage in with your relative that can enable him to share his special identity and knowledge. You may wish to produce a video of your relative recalling past experiences and narrating family history no one else knows about. Not only will it affirm his importance to the family, it is a lasting gift only he can give you.

Sharing the Care

When I am asked to make a decision for my loved one that she is now unable to make for herself, I do what I think she would do if she were able. I remember back to conversations with her. I consider feelings she expressed in the past. I try to recall if there were similar experiences she had to deal with before and what actions she took.

Consider this: When the family is concerned with some aspect of the care or has a complaint, the family spokesperson should be the only one to contact the facility. The designated person should know the appropriate staff member to contact and do so professionally and tactfully. It is a good idea to do it in writing as well as in person.

Sharing the Care

I am emotionally involved with my loved one. I try to maintain the same relationship we have always had, but some changes have occurred. However, the surroundings and the present situation should not keep us from enjoying many of the things we have shared in the past—including our respect for each other's place in the family structure.

Consider this: Caregiving responsibilities and circumstances can cause necessary changes in relationships and the roles we play. The delicate balance of your position in the family may be altered, but the emotional connection can remain and everyone's dignity maintained.

Sharing the Care

My loved one was always an inspiration to our family. Her faith uplifted all of us. Her smile was a ray of sunshine on dark days. Her words encouraged us when we were down. I am grateful for her spiritual strength and I look for ways to add hope to her days.

Consider this: A large-print copy of the Bible is a thoughtful gift for residents of care facilities. The Bible is also available on audiocassettes in almost every language. Some family caregivers print scriptures and inspirational messages and place them on their relative's bulletin board or by the bed. This can be uplifting for staff as well as residents!

Sharing the Care

My loved one repeats things. I listen. I practice patience. Sometimes I bring a younger family member with me who loves to ask him to retell favorite stories. My mind often wanders—while they have a wonderful time!

Consider this: Your relative is most likely surrounded by people who share the same kind of memories. Bring some antique items in when you visit. Seeing and holding the memorabilia will most likely spark conversation among your relative and other residents. They'll enjoy themselves and you'll probably get a wonderful history lesson!

Sharing the Care

Some conversations with my loved one are difficult for both of us. There are important issues that have to be discussed while she is able. She initiates some of these discussions. She needs to talk and make her desires known. I listen and reassure her I will do everything possible to carry out her wishes.

Consider this: Knowing funeral plans and preferences ahead of time can be reassuring for your relative and you. Elderly people are often quite definite about their feelings. Your relative may want a say in where she is to be buried and what clothing she is to wear. She might even know what she wants written on her tombstone and what kind of service she'd like. By making her wishes known, she is helping her family.

Sharing the Care

Visits are not always remembered by my loved one. He often complains he never sees me or other family members. I don't stop coming. I am reinforced of the importance of our visits. Maybe it's his way of telling me how much being with me means to him!

Consider this: On your next visit, try writing a note before you leave. Put the date on it and tell a little something about your visit. Mention what you did together and what kind of things you talked about. State that you will return again soon and sign the note. Give the note to a nurse or aide and ask them to show it to your relative whenever he asks about you or complains that you haven't been there. Some families use a visitors' log. Each visitor makes an entry. It's kept in a prominent place in their relative's room.

Sharing the Care

I am an important link to my loved one's identity and self-worth. I call her by name. I give her sincere compliments. I remember and respect her likes and dislikes. I do whatever I can to help her maintain her dignity and self-esteem.

Consider this: One caregiver knew it was important to her relative to dress nicely and to be color-coordinated. The caregiver arranged all the clothes in the closet by colors and matching outfits. It made it easier for the aides who dressed her relative and it helped her relative feel good about her appearance.

Sharing the Care

I've been a child. I've experienced adolescence. Now I'm an adult. But I don't know what old age is like. I haven't had the losses most elderly people have. Family members, friends, hearing, eyesight, mobility, financial independence, and the ability to make decisions for yourself are among the losses older people suffer. I can't begin to know what it is like. I can, however, treat my loved one with the compassion and respect he deserves.

Consider this: If your relative has always attended a church or synagogue and is unable to do so now, he may be missing the people he fellowshipped with there. Ask the church or synagogue secretary to put him on their mailing list. He'll enjoy the news regarding members he knows. Do the same thing for clubs and organizations he has belonged to.

Sharing the Care

I've become more creative in the ways I express my love and concern for my loved one. I strive for quality in our visits. I may not be spending as much time with her as I did in the past, but the time I do spend with her is loving and nurturing. I am able to focus on her and at the same time oversee her care.

Consider this: Join your relative for a meal once in a while. A day's notice to the facility is probably sufficient. Your relative will love having your company and be proud for her friends to see you dining with her. You'll be able to experience what her meals and mealtime are like first-hand.

Sharing the Care

Kindness, consideration, and compassion always soothe and nurture the human spirit. The emotional needs for such things don't diminish with age or illness. In fact, they may grow stronger. Professional caregivers are providing my relative's physical needs now, but for the most part he looks to his family for his emotional needs.

Consider this: Even if your relative has dementia or a severe hearing problem, don't talk about him as if he isn't in the room. He probably hears and understands more than you think he does. Discourage other family members, nurses, and aides from talking about him in his presence. Simple politeness is always in order.

Sharing the Care

Even though my loved one can't do some of the things he used to, he still enjoys doing many things. There are numerous activities he looks forward to. He isn't bored.

Consider this: Hobbies and interests can be continued in the care facility setting. If reading good books or the classics is an interest still enjoyed by your relative, ask him if there are certain books you can bring him. Antique and used bookstores are excellent sources of hard to find older books. If reading is difficult due to fading eyesight, look in regular book stores and the public library for his favorites in large-print or on audio cassettes.

Sharing the Care

I am thankful for a facility staffed by competent, caring professionals. The attention, the understanding, and the love they show our relative is valued by our whole family.

Consider this: Families of residents often show their appreciation to staff by bringing in candy, fruit, or ordering pizzas for everyone. If you do this, be sure to include each shift. The night shift usually gets left out because the families don't know them. They deserve to be acknowledged and remembered, too!

Sharing the Care

My loved one always enjoyed being a hostess. She delighted in entertaining family and friends in her home. This doesn't have to change because the surroundings have changed. She is just as gracious when I visit her in this home. I let her know I enjoy her hospitality.

Consider this: Your relative should feel comfortable having guests in her new home. Many care facilities provide lovely family rooms for the residents and their guests. Often they have a special room, which can be reserved for private parties. Most facilities encourage residents to entertain and will cooperate in any way they can.

Sharing the Care

No matter how much we love each other, my relative and I have never seen things eye-to-eye. In fact, our relationship has gone from bad to worse. As he ages, I feel guilty about my feelings because age makes him seem vulnerable and defenseless. I'm trying to mend some fences, but I'm not making much progress.

Consider this: If your relationship with your relative has been difficult, don't expect miracles just because he has aged and moved into a care facility. If you have been the primary caregiver, things may improve because you are no longer doing the day-to-day caregiving chores. You may be freer to relax and enjoy each other now. You might both wish to make an effort to improve your relationship. Try talking about it with him.

Sharing the Care

My visits are a time of enjoying my loved one, but there are also some caregiving chores I perform during visits. It's part of my role as overseer. I don't let any of these tasks appear to be burdens. I do them because I care. I never want my loved one to think she is a burden to me.

Consider this: Go through your relative's clothes periodically. Make sure her personal items are in good shape. Replace or repair things when necessary. Whether you do her laundry or the facility does, always keep a laundry pen handy. Mark new items with her name and room number. Keep identification on old items legible. You and the facility should both have an accurate up-to-date list of her clothing and other items. Remember to add all gifts and new purchases to both lists!

Sharing the Care

I'm good to myself. I have interests and a life of my own. My identity is important. I tell my relative about my life and my activities. Talking about what I am involved in often triggers memories and conversations of similar things he has done.

Consider this: If you have recently returned from a trip, share your photos or slides with your relative. They can be a good discussion topic. Ask him about past trips he has taken. Discuss the modes of transportation he used. Consider sharing videos of your trips with all the residents. Ask the staff if you can show travel videos on the large television screen in the lounge.

Sharing the Care

There is a sensitive balance in every family relationship. Roles and positions within our family are respected. I am, however, aware that age, illness, and circumstances beyond our control can upset the usual balance. I may have been thrust into a new role that I am not all together comfortable with. I try not to over-step boundaries or appear controlling.

Consider this: Your relative's room or suite is her home and should be treated as such. Ask her permission before changing something, putting up decorations, or removing anything.

Sharing the Care

My loved one was an integral part of his community. His knowledge made him a leader. There wasn't a subject he couldn't discuss. The world doesn't have to pass him by just because he moves a little slower today. I can help him stay informed and I will learn from his experience and wisdom. He may provide me with a better perspective.

Consider this: If newspaper print is too small for your relative to read, offer to read the paper to him. If you are unable to do this, many facilities have a group activity session every morning in which a staff member or volunteer reads the local paper out loud for the residents. Many articles become topics of conversation between the residents. If appropriate, consider arranging daily newspaper delivery for your relative.

Sharing the Care

I encourage other members of our family to stay in touch with our loved one. If they live out of town, letters and occasional phone calls mean so much to her. I let her share their news with me—even if I already know about it.

Consider this: Many residents of care facilities have telephones by their beds. If your relative cannot initiate calls or you are worried about others using the phone, see if a phone can be installed that only takes incoming calls. If your relative has trouble reading her mail, read it to her. The activity can be a pleasant time for both of you.

Sharing the Care

I quietly observe the faces of the staff when I visit. They tell me a lot about the quality of care my loved one is receiving. Their faces reveal more than their voices do. I can tell if they are preoccupied or under too much stress.

Consider this: You will probably know if the care facility is under-staffed. If they hurry the residents, your relative may not be getting the care or attention you want him to have. If the staff acts crabby and upset with each other, that attitude may carry on to interchanges with the residents. Don't go looking for trouble, but be aware of the overall attitude of the staff. Keep in mind, everyone has a bad day once in a while but observance of continually unpleasant expressions or behaviors of staff members is cause for concern.

Sharing the Care

Sometimes my loved one asks me to take her home. She even asks if she can go to my home with me. I feel sad for her. I also experience guilt because I can't take her home and she can't live with me. I just tell her I wish I could, but I can't.

Consider this: If your relative has dementia, asking for home could mean a number of things. She may be searching for her younger self or a place that is more familiar. If she were home again, she might still continue to ask to go home. Work with the staff to help her feel as secure as possible. Surround her with familiar things, love, and reassurance.

Sharing the Care

Our family still talks about our relative's cooking. I encourage her to pass favorite recipes on to us! In trying to help her feel at home, the staff and I realize that one of the most important and familiar parts of home for her is the kitchen.

Consider this: Most facilities have a small kitchen that can be used by residents and their families. Encourage your relative to partake of any cooking activities the staff provides for the residents. Use the kitchen with her to prepare favorite recipes together. Share the results with other residents and the staff or send to family members as gifts from your relative stating it's from her kitchen. Be sure to include a copy of the recipe—just the way she always made it!

Sharing the Care

The way I perceive the care facility and the way I conduct myself when I am there is not only important for me, it may have an effect on others who observe me. If I see it as depressing or an end-of-the-line aspect of life, those around me and my loved one may begin to think of it that way, too. My attitude is a very contagious thing!

Consider this: Adult family members are role models to the younger members in a family. Without realizing it, you could be helping form opinions and views the young people who look up to you may carry for a lifetime. If you treat everyone in the care facility with love and respect and see the facility as a home with a heart, they will too.

Sharing the Care

My best efforts cannot halt the aging process. Aging is a part of living. I cannot stop it, avoid it, or deny it. Like everything else life hands us, it is the manner in which we face aging in ourselves and others that is important.

Consider this: Elderly skin is more vulnerable than young skin. It is thin and tears easily. You may need to pad sharp corners on furniture. Also when wheeling your relative's wheelchair, remind her not to rest her arms with her elbows sticking out too far. This will help avoid bumping or scraping her skin.

Sharing the Care

I encourage my loved one to continue to do the things he does well and enjoys doing. Sometimes he needs me to remind him of his talents and interests. He doesn't initiate things as spontaneously as he used to—so now it's one of the things I help him with. Whenever I suggest an old activity he enjoyed in the past and can still do, his face lights up and he joins right in!

Consider this: Most facilities have pianos in their lounge or activity room. Playing the piano is a skill not easily forgotten. Many dementia patients still play and enjoy the piano long after other skills are lost. Some bedridden patients are able to play on portable electronic keyboards.

Sharing the Care

I'm not afraid to talk about real issues. There are some things my loved one and I have to discuss. We don't put them off. We don't put each other off. We respect what the other deems important.

Consider this: You may find your relative sharing personal medical issues with you. Elderly people are often more open or preoccupied with things we'd rather not hear about. But, as a caregiver you are involved and these conversations may alert you to a care or medical problem, which might otherwise go, undetected.

Sharing the Care

When my loved one is troubled or sad, I just try to love her through it. I can't always make her feel better, but I can listen and tell her I understand. I validate her right to feel. I don't make judgments on her feelings. If she is obsessing or constantly repeating her woes, I try to introduce more pleasant conversation for both our sakes!

Consider this: You are not responsible for your relative's feelings or outlook on life. Expect some grieving on her part. She is experiencing the natural losses old age brings. She may have steps to walk through or some old unfinished business she needs to deal with. You might be able to help in some areas, but remember she's got a lot of years, wisdom, and experience going for her.

Sharing the Care

No matter what kind of visit my loved one and I have, I try to end each visit on an upbeat note. A pleasant ending should help both of us look forward to the next time we're together. Even if his memory is shaky or fading, I'll remember the visit better if it ends well!

Consider this: The tone of visits can be set or changed more easily by you. You can bring in news or tales of interesting things you encounter, participate in, or hear about. Your life is most likely filled with more diversity than your relative's. Sharing the world outside the care facility with your loved one can be something you both look forward to.

Sharing the Care

I know I am doing the best I can for my loved one and part of that is taking good care of myself. I continue to enjoy regular vacations and recreation. When I go out of town, I let the staff know how to reach me in an extreme emergency. I also arrange for another family member or friend to be available locally.

Consider this: If you are the primary caregiver or family member who spends the most time with your loved one, ask other family members or friends to drop in and see her occasionally while you are gone. You have probably made friends or become acquainted with family members of other residents. They may take a little extra time to check on and visit with your relative in your absence. If convenient, send postcards to your relative and the staff.

Sharing the Care

I've always avoided power struggles. The present circumstances and the position I have been put in often distresses me. I am forced to make important decisions. I have power I'd rather not have. Sometimes my loved one disagrees with me and I am uncomfortable in this role. He seems so vulnerable. I seem so powerful.

Consider this: When your relative appears upset with you, it is more likely he is upset with the circumstances and the things he can no longer control. He may also be losing some of the ability to express himself adequately. When he gets angry, you get the brunt of it. Understanding and level thinking on your part will be more appreciated than you'll ever know.

Sharing the Care

Accusing or blaming someone for something is judgmental and it puts them on the defensive. I don't like it when someone treats me that way. I'll make sure I don't jump to conclusions and attack people.

Consider this: There will be times when you are upset with someone in the facility or some policy of the facility. Or, there may even be an upsetting incident involving a resident. Possessions sometimes disappear. Residents may occasionally fight with one another. Be sure to check everything out calmly and thoroughly. A solution will be more easily and quickly arrived at if you approach the situation with a non-blaming attitude.

Sharing the Care

I respect the staff and administration. I don't bother them with petty things or constantly ask them questions. They have a job to do. Alternatively, I have a job to do, too. I am the overall manager of my loved one's care. His care is ultimately my responsibility.

Consider this: You are as much an authority on your relative's care as the facility administration and personnel—probably more. Don't be afraid to ask questions that are important to you, such as how often your relative gets a full bath or shower. You can request to see menus for the week or month. Question the staff, pharmacist, or physician if you have a concern or are not being kept up-to-date on your relative's medications.

Sharing the Care

Why is it I can carry on a twenty-minute conversation with another resident, but after five minutes with my relative we find ourselves sitting in silence? Have we said it all? Or, have we forgotten how to communicate with each other?

Consider this: Sometimes closeness is more important than words. Your presence is probably very important to your loved one. And, remember if he has a form of dementia, communication will be hindered. If he is not confused, and the silences bother you, ask him if he is concerned. Role reversal may have caused communication between the two of you to be temporarily awkward. Life-changes often bring changes in communication. Learning new ways may be the answer.

Sharing the Care

I can't always do what my loved one wants. I have to evaluate his needs. He doesn't like some of the care he requires. He doesn't always understand. Or, maybe he does, but he shows his anger and frustrations by arguing with me. I don't try to explain. I tell him I understand how he feels.

Consider this: Don't take on guilt feelings because your relative has certain care needs he objects to. You have probably discussed them with him. Going over them again and trying to convince him something is necessary can be futile. Try to make sure his dignity is maintained as much as possible in every situation. You're doing the best you can for him—and, you're doing a great job!

Sharing the Care

Reminiscing is a wonderful way my loved one and I communicate. I encourage her to share memories. I show interest and ask details. I thank her for the gift of sharing history and often forgotten values with me.

Consider this: Try to connect the past to the present. Compare yesterday's pictures of town landmarks with pictures taken recently. Ask your relative questions about ways of doing things long ago. Share with her new ways they are done today. The exchange and comparisons can be interesting and fun for both of you.

Sharing the Care

I am concerned when I see my loved one sad and withdrawing from other people or activities. It's not consistent with his personality and I don't feel it is an inevitable part of aging. His outlook on life is usually positive, so something must be going on that we need to look into.

Consider this: Sometimes we accept sadness, sleeping problems, withdrawal, or forgetfulness as a normal result of the aging process when they may be symptoms of depression. Make sure you mention any concerns you have to the staff and certainly to your relative's doctor. Depression in the elderly is not uncommon and can usually be treated successfully.

Sharing the Care

Having something to look forward to is always fun. This doesn't diminish with age. I realize my visits are among the things my loved one looks forward to. We've talked about spring and we're both anxious to see the trees bud and the migrating birds return.

Consider this: The fresh smell of outdoors can be very refreshing to someone who has spent months inside the care facility. As soon as the weather permits, encourage strolls outside together when you visit. Point out emerging green plants and birds building nests. Take time and breathe in the fresh spring air!

Sharing the Care

My loved one is trying his hand at painting. It is something he has always wanted to do. I'm so glad he's doing it now. I encourage him and look forward to seeing his work each time I visit. I've asked him if he'll paint something especially for me. It's a gift I will cherish.

Consider this: Everyone likes to have a sense of accomplishment. If your relative needs a boost in self-confidence or a new interest, be supportive in the things that seem to stimulate him. Crafts and hobbies usually go a long way in promoting self-esteem. There can be a shine in the golden years!

Sharing the Care

It's important for my relative to know her life has purpose. I make a point of talking to her about the things that are significant to her. I recognize her strengths and accomplishments. I thank her for the things she has done for me. I let her know she has a special place in our family. Her life has meaning to all of us.

Consider this: If your relative has encouraged and nurtured you in the past, it will be easy for you to validate her worth. But, if it's difficult for you, try using phrases such as, "I'd like to hear more about the time you . . ." or "I admire the way you . . ." You'll be amazed how this will help her self-confidence and also enhance your communication with her.

Sharing the Care

Today is a special day for my loved one. We have planned an appropriate celebration. He doesn't like surprises. He enjoys taking part in the preparations. It's his day and his home. We've worked together to make it a festive, yet comfortable time for all.

Consider this: Be considerate of your relative's abilities when you wrap presents for him. Solid brightly colored paper can be seen more easily than paper with small designs or tiny written messages. Loosely tie the packages with wide ribbons or heavy yarn. Don't knot the ribbon or yarn. Avoid using tape. Your thoughtfulness will help make the day more enjoyable for him and he'll not be embarrassed by needing help to open his gifts.

Sharing the Care

I try not to let my loved one's health problems and limitations depress me. I am doing everything I can for her—so is the care facility staff.

Consider this: When someone is in pain, it's better to put your hand under theirs, rather than to hold their hand. Don't put yours on top where it may be too heavy for them or where you may inadvertently exert too much pressure. Sitting next to someone who is ill is more considerate than standing. They won't strain as much to see you and you will appear more comforting sitting near them. Suggest that nurses give medications from a sitting position, rather than standing over your relative.

Sharing the Care

I notice that my loved one and other residents smile a lot whenever there is a child in the room. They delight in seeing the fresh beauty and joy in a child's face. They eagerly join a child's laughter. A spirit of health and hope is revived.

Consider this: Many nursery schools and child day care programs make regular visits to adult care facilities. The young and the elderly love each other's company. They enjoy signing, dancing, talking, and laughing together. Shared crafts, stories, and ice cream cones are often a part of their get-togethers.

Sharing the Care

For the most part, the staff members are dedicated workers. I appreciate the care and time they give my loved one. I tell them so. Some in particular have become very important people in my relative's life.

Consider this: Often residents and their family members want to give cards or small gifts to special staff members on their birthdays. Check with the staff administrator first, as there may be a policy against doing so. Also make sure it won't cause bad feelings on the part of other workers. It might be a good idea to remember the birthdays of everyone who works closely with your relative. In that case, cards with a personalized note of thanks may be sufficient.

Sharing the Care

Part of overseeing my loved one's care and comfort is making sure his clothes are comfortable. Changes in weight can require changes in clothing. Health issues can determine needs in appropriate apparel. Safety is also a factor to be considered when purchasing his wardrobe and accessories.

Consider this: Having the proper attire seems to be a necessary and ongoing part of life. Washable slip-on canvas shoes with rubber soles are very practical, safe, and comfortable. Velcro fastenings are easier than laces on shoes or buttons on clothes. Soft or baggy clothing is always a relief for those who spend a great deal of time sitting. Apparel that is easily removed and loose fitting is best for dealing with incontinence. Well-made machine-washable garments are a must for anyone residing in a care facility!

Sharing the Care

Music has always been a part of my loved one's life. Although she no longer plays an instrument, listening to music is an important component of her world. She should not be detached from her connection with this beautiful expression of life. I do everything I can to help keep her musical interests alive.

Consider this: Make sure the staff knows of her love of music. Ask them to inform her of all musical activities or presentations the facility offers. Bring in tapes of favorite recordings to listen to. Let her know of upcoming musical programs or specials on television. If appropriate and convenient, attend community symphonic performances and concerts together. And, don't forget, music boxes always make great gifts!

Sharing the Care

Every visit with my relative is a time of learning. By being attentive and asking him questions about the past, I learn more about our family history. I never had quality time alone with him before. I'm enjoying this special privilege of really getting to know him. In the process I'm learning more about myself and my roots.

Consider this: Your visits can be a time you look forward to. In the quiet person-to-person setting you can get to know and respect each other as individuals—as well as reinforce the family love and connection. It's a wonderful opportunity for both of you to discover or rediscover the real people behind the faces in those family portraits.

Sharing the Care

I let my loved one feel her feelings.
Feelings are not right or wrong—they just are.
If someone is not allowed to own their
feelings or they aren't free to express them,
they can't work through them. Often they
disguise them in complaints or difficult
behavior.

Consider this: Don't put your relative's
feelings down or force her to defend them.
Listen to her and trust that she will
successfully come through any feelings she
may have such as grief, displacement, or
loneliness. We continue to feel, grow, and
change no matter what age we are.
Minimizing someone's feelings or trying to
make them feel better doesn't allow them the
freedom to move on.

Sharing the Care

My loved one looks at aging as being normal wear and tear. He realizes that occasional forgetfulness is not memory loss. He accepts the natural aging process he is experiencing. He knows his limitations. For the most part, he recognizes what is good for him and what is not.

Consider this: Diminished hearing, fading vision, or the fear of falling, can make excursions outside the care facility difficult for your relative. He is accustomed to the surroundings he lives in. Being away from familiar landmarks could be upsetting, uncomfortable, or even dangerous for him. Understand if he is reluctant to go on facility offered tours—or even trips to family members' homes.

Sharing the Care

I know the value of support groups. Sharing between members is an important part of getting through difficult times in our lives. I'm fortunate to meet with others who are experiencing the same life-changes I am.

Consider this: Many care facilities offer support group meetings for the family members of their residents. If yours does not, look into forming one. Or, perhaps your local council on aging or other community services may be able to direct you to an appropriate group. Caregivers in your church or neighborhood might be interested in getting together. Overseeing the care of a family member can be exhausting and overwhelming without the support and mutual understanding of other caregivers.

Sharing the Care

If I find I have an unpleasant feeling during or after visits with my loved one, I need to discover the reason for those feelings. Am I sad or guilt-ridden? Am I harboring any resentments? What can I do to work through the feelings?

Consider this: Your own emotional well being is of utmost importance. If you cannot get to the bottom of your uneasiness, talk to someone you trust. A counselor, a close friend, or a member of the clergy may be able to help you. It is not unusual to feel stressed in your situation. A caring professional will suggest ways to deal with your feelings appropriately and ways to ease your stress.

Sharing the Care

I don't let my loved one be compromised. If I believe her rights are being infringed upon, I talk to the administrator in a non-threatening and cooperative manner. If after discussing the matter, I feel it is not being resolved to my loved one's best care interests, the services of an ombudsman are called for.

Consider this: The ombudsman services work for residents, family members, and facility employees to resolve problems, the resolution of which will improve resident care. Ombudsmen are to thoroughly investigate and attempt to resolve any concerns they receive. They also work with all interested groups to define issues relative to long-term care facilities. They often work with such groups to implement needed changes in legislation and regulations.

Sharing the Care

It's very difficult to see my loved one ill. The staff is wonderful with her. I am grateful to them for the care and gentleness they show. They are trained in ways I am not, but together we help keep her as comfortable as possible.

Consider this: When someone is ill or bedridden in a care facility, aides and family members are usually with the patients more than doctors or nurses. If your relative is ill, ask the nurses for suggestions as to how you can best help your relative. Keeping someone's mouth fresh and moist, offering water or crushed ice often, applying a cool washcloth to her face, and keeping the bed linen wrinkle-free are among the many things you can do.

Sharing the Care

There are times my loved one just needs a new interest. Perhaps a little spark that pushes him to think about something from a new angle—something that encourages him to stretch a little and consider things beyond himself.

Consider this: There are many forms of art therapy that can renew interests and revitalize the way things are seen. Art expression can be fun. Viewing different forms of art, such as paintings and sculptures and then choosing colors to express the feelings they evoke is an excellent activity. Discussion of art or writing words that come to mind upon studying certain art pieces can be thought provoking and interesting. No opinions or views are wrong!

Sharing the Care

My loved one has physical problems that necessitate his residing in the care facility, but his mental and social abilities are fine. He's able to assume and perform his role as an elder in the family, the community, and society. He's a valuable human resource. He has experienced, coped with, and survived a lot during his life. He is a big help to others going through life-changing happenings.

Consider this: Our elders have something very special to give. Even those with dementia often retain talents and social skills that can be shared. Many churches and community organizations meet regularly with residents of care facilities—not just to make visits to the elderly, but to learn from them how they've dealt with things such as the loss of a spouse or child, retirement, career changes, serious illnesses, and more.

Sharing the Care

The first day of May used to be a special day of celebration. Children danced around Maypoles. Homemade baskets filled with spring flowers were placed on neighbors' front porches. It was a joyful day!

Consider this: A May basket will be appreciated by your elderly relative—especially if the flowers come from your garden. You might want to ask the administrator if you can plant a flowering garden on the facility grounds. Select flowers that can be enjoyed and picked by the staff and the residents. Plant a variety to insure flowering over many months. Include some that will bloom into autumn.

Sharing the Care

I notice a certain degree of family withdrawal. Some of our family members choose not to visit our relative. A number of excuses and reasons are given.

Consider this: It's not unusual for some family members to have difficulties accepting the placement of a relative in a long-term care facility. Unreal expectations, guilt, denial, and the inability to face aging or failing health can all contribute to avoidance by some family members. If you find this occurring in individuals in your family, encourage them to discuss their feelings, fears, and concerns with someone they are comfortable with. Hopefully, they can overcome these obstacles and begin to be a part of their relative's life again.

Sharing the Care

I frequently offer my loved one fresh water—and I join her. It's something we do together, rather than me treating her like a patient. Sometimes I bring fresh lemon or lime to enhance it. I notice if her mouth is dry or moist when I arrive. If it is always dry, I remind the staff she may need their involvement to drink water throughout the day. Just because there is a glass and pitcher near her, doesn't mean she'll drink it by herself.

Consider this: Liquid intake is very important. Dementia patients in particular need to be encouraged to drink lots of water. They won't always do it on their own. Cutting down on liquids will not prevent incontinence. Too little liquid intake can make the urine more concentrated and cause bladder irritation and problems.

Sharing the Care

I've observed how the residents support one another. Often it is done without words. A smile, a pat on the back, or a nod between friends is reassuring. Strong bonds have been formed.

Consider this: Being with and seeing the same people every day can be comforting and reassuring. Consistency is especially important for residents with dementia. Most facilities encourage activities in small groups. Make sure your relative sits with one or two close friends at mealtimes.

Sharing the Care

I still use most of the skills I learned and practiced when I cared for my loved one at home. Often I help the staff by sharing my acquired solutions to specific problems and challenges. I offer help and suggestions cheerfully—I don't act like I know it all. I'm still learning too!

Consider this: If there is space, consider putting a rocking chair in your relative's room. Rocking is an especially good activity for anyone who is restless or tends to pace a lot. For someone with Alzheimer's disease it may help prevent wandering or provide some relief if sundowning is a problem. Bringing in a familiar rocking chair from your relative's home can be a very welcome addition to his room.

Sharing the Care

My loved one likes small, varied activities. He also seems to enjoy some personal quiet-time and individual projects. I look for new ideas and small endeavors that interest him.

Consider this: Adult coloring books can be found in museum gift shops, art galleries, and in specialty shops. They can also be purchased from some organizations such as the Audubon Society. They make great gifts for care facility residents. Often non-toxic colored pens work better than crayons and are more appropriate for adults.

Sharing the Care

The staff and I have a wonderful understanding. We agree not to believe what my loved one says about the other. When she tells the staff I have stolen her belongings and she tells me the staff or other residents have taken everything she had, we just help her look for missing items and don't get into how they disappeared!

Consider this: Things just seem to get misplaced in congregate living conditions. Individuals suffering from Alzheimer's disease or a related disorder often hide or lose items without realizing it. Some residents may innocently take things that don't belong to them. Suspicion is often a factor to contend with in residents with dementia. And, no matter how well run the facility's laundry is, clothing will get lost or inadvertently placed in the wrong rooms.

Sharing the Care

My attitude about anything in life usually improves when I get involved. This concept certainly applies to the care facility. If I choose to be an outsider who only comes to visit my relative, that's my privilege. But, when I make an effort to interact with the residents, the staff, and other families—we all benefit!

Consider this: Your family or the facility family council can have great fun looking for, purchasing, and restoring a player piano for the residents' lounge. Many hours of enjoyment can be had by all!

Sharing the Care

I mention my loved one's life accomplishments often when we talk. These recollections not only set the path to wonderful reminiscing, they also strengthen the bond between us and retain his feelings of self-worth. I'm a good listener and I ask questions that genuinely interest me. My inquiries also provide opportunities for him to tell me things I didn't know—even if the subject is one we have discussed before!

Consider this: There are specialty magazines that focus on days gone-by. They usually contain old advertisements, nostalgic articles, and quaint stories. Old Sears and Roebuck catalogs are also available. There are a number of publications that can help you encourage reminiscent conversations with your elderly relative.

Sharing the Care

It's good for my loved one to function as independently as possible. I encourage him to dress himself and to do as much of his own personal care as he can. He may require help with some things, but there are still many things he can do. He has never wanted anyone fussing over him or waiting on him.

Consider this: Many people who are confined to wheelchairs can "walk" while sitting, if the footrests are moved out of the way. They become quite mobile by moving their feet and using their arms and hands to push or pull when they come in contact with a door handle, a wall railing, or furniture. Be sure the wheels are locked for safety when the staff transfers your relative to or from the wheelchair. Also the brakes should be used when his wheelchair is positioned at the table for meals or other stationary activities.

Sharing the Care

Sometimes my loved one has trouble expressing herself. She says some things I know she doesn't really mean. I listen to her comments and try to see behind them to discover what is really bothering her. When I make an effort to truly hear her and not interject my reactions, I usually get to the root of the problem.

Consider this: Try mirroring your relative's feelings. You can do this by being a good listener and then saying, "it sounds like you ..." or "is this what you're feeling?" This method of feeding back her feelings shows that you genuinely care and want to understand. You are not judging her feelings or taking a stand of your own regarding her comments.

Sharing the Care

The human touch is important to all of us. Whenever I am with my loved one I reach out and touch him. I hug him when I arrive and when I leave. We often hold hands when we walk together. I give him reassuring pats whenever I can. I need them as much as he does!

Consider this: We often worry that our relatives won't get the physical contact they need when they live in a care facility. Group activities such as dancing can provide human contact. Sitting on a sofa next to another resident often helps. Observe the way the aides touch your relative when they care for him. If you do not feel they are gentle enough, tell them in a nice way. Also be sure to tell them when you appreciate the tender way they treat him.

Sharing the Care

Letting go has always been a difficult thing for me. But, the times I have let go of my need to control have usually been the times I have benefited most and things have worked out the best.

Consider this: Former primary caregivers usually fear they will lose control over the care of their loved ones when placement in a care facility is made. What they usually find is they have not lost control. They lose much of the stress they felt previously. There is relief and comfort in knowing they are part of a team. Care chores are now shared. Family caregivers still retain a responsible position without the day-to-day physical and emotional stresses they experienced before.

Sharing the Care

I try to be present when my loved one's physician visits her, but I can't always be there or know when he is expected. If there is something I am concerned about or have a question about, I leave a note for the doctor with the head nurse. If he does not address my concerns, I call him.

Consider this: Most doctors are involved with curing people. Many family members of long-term care facility residents feel their relatives are neglected by their previous physicians. Some families have replaced them with doctors who practice geriatric medicine. They specialize in the elderly and the unique aspects of aging. Also the effects of dementia and Alzheimer's disease are more apt to be understood and addressed by geriatric and neurological specialists.

Sharing the Care

Special days hold special meanings for all of us. The elderly treasure traditions. There is much significance in family holidays. Our family makes a point of including residents who may not have family or whose families live a distance away and are unable to attend the facility get-togethers.

Consider this: Mother's Day can be acknowledged and celebrated in many different ways. A formal tea with families and staff members hosting the event is very popular. Another successful function is a luncheon and style show held in the facility's formal dining room. Residents, daughters, and granddaughters enjoy modeling the clothing. Style shows are often hosted by local stores and the attendees can make purchases the day of the event.

Sharing the Care

My loved one is a survivor! He wouldn't have lived so long if he weren't. I admire his strength of body and character. I sometimes find myself quietly studying him to see exactly what that strength consists of. Where does it come from? Do I have it too? Is it learned or is it genetic?

Consider this: Some people just seem to take life in their stride. They are usually people who possess a good sense of humor and face things realistically. Whatever confronts them does not overcome them. They don't tend to be worriers. They are usually interested in other people and in the world around them. A lot can be learned from survivors!

Sharing the Care

My loved one can no longer communicate with me in words. We are learning new ways of telling each other our feelings and our needs. Body language has become very important. Facial expressions, nods, and touching have all taken on new significance.

Consider this: Family members are often concerned as to how they would know if their non-speaking relative is in pain. This is often a factor when dealing with advanced Alzheimer's disease. There are a number of ways pain might be expressed. Moaning or screaming out are fairly obvious signs. Wiggling toes and clenching fists are others. Some people breath in and out deeply and heavily when in pain. Restless or fitful sleeping could also indicate pain.

Sharing the Care

Some things just can't be avoided. Placing blame for certain occurrences is pointless. If I can't change a situation, I can try adjusting my perception of it. How it affects me and how I see it are within my control.

Consider this: Residents often wrap their own dentures in napkins, handkerchiefs, or Kleenex. They can be inadvertently placed on the dinner table or tray and tossed out with meal leftovers. Sometimes they are rolled up in the bed linens and vanish in the laundry. Hearing aides and eyeglasses can be easily misplaced. Try to have identification on these items. Ask the administration what their position is regarding the facility's responsibility. Some states have specific laws spelling out what must be done to protect such belongings.

Sharing the Care

I expect the environment my loved one inhabits to be safe. Safety is an important aspect of his care. He cannot live alone and I trust the care facility to provide for him in a responsibly compassionate and reasonably secure manner.

Consider this: Most facilities have adequate provisions for safety. Handrails should be installed along hallways. Fire alarms and clearly marked exits are a must. A system should be in operation to prevent wandering outside by residents with dementia. Medications must be monitored and administered properly. If you observe a hazardous practice by the staff or an aspect of the physical building you feel is unsafe, point it out to the administration. Approach the subject in a non-threatening, yet concerned fashion.

Sharing the Care

My loved one is very gracious and lovely. She always has been. That has never changed. She is a beautiful lady. I tell her so!

Consider this: Although it is impractical to give your relative expensive gifts, there are many feminine things she may appreciate. A new hairbrush, fresh lipstick, powder, and rouge may be welcomed. Soft-scented cologne or body lotion is always a nice addition. Music boxes with figurines on top are entertaining and their tunes can be great tools for reminiscing. Some ladies love dollhouses. Rearranging the tiny furniture can provide hours of delight for previous homemakers.

Sharing the Care

Sometimes big is better. Because of the changes in my loved one's eyesight, his physical condition, or his overall abilities, the larger something is, the easier it is to deal with and the more comfortable it may be. I keep this in mind when I bring him new items or suggest new activities.

Consider this: A clock with large numbers may be appreciated by your relative. Loose-fitting men's sweaters and ladies' shawls make dressing easier for arthritis sufferers. Large playing cards for games and solitaire are easier to see and handle. If you bring in a new board game, rewrite the directions in large bold print. It's a good idea to do this on a stiff piece of cardboard that won't be lost easily. You might want to tape it to the box.

Sharing the Care

I'm not afraid to say no. The things I do for my loved one are by choice—not obligation. If I give in to unreasonable demands, I am not being fair to either one of us. We have an adult relationship and I plan to keep it that way. Mutual respect is a necessary part of our relationship no matter what the circumstances.

Consider this: The care facility is an extension of your love and concern. It is there to help you with the care of your relative. You should be under less stress and better able to enjoy your relative now. If you feel he is depending on you too much or asking the impossible of you, talk to the staff about it. You might even be able to discuss it with him. Maybe he doesn't realize that his demands on you are unrealistic and cause you distress.

Sharing the Care

Change is inevitable. Not only does my loved one change, the facility changes from time to time—and so do I! Some changes are good. Some are not so good. Some can be controlled. Some cannot. My resistance to change can cause me problems. I need to accept the changes that are out of my hands.

Consider this: Turnover in care facility personnel is certainly inevitable and something you will have to live with. Unfortunately, the wages for aides are notoriously low. If something more lucrative comes along for them, they often change to another facility or another line of work. You may find a change in the staff on weekends if the facility has to hire help from an agency. Occasionally there will be policy changes that you don't expect and can do nothing about.

Sharing the Care

My loved one was always athletic and physically active. Due to circumstances beyond his control, he is now limited in the type and the amount of exercise he can participate in. He enjoys talking about sports with me. I make sure he still receives the sports publications he has subscribed to for years.

Consider this: Depending on your relative's physical capabilities, there are a number of good exercises you can do with him. Marching in place, stretching, and arm or neck movements are popular. Facial exercises are beneficial. Try raising your eyebrows, wrinkling your noses, and winking at each other. You'll probably both end up laughing—perhaps the best exercise of all!

Sharing the Care

Some of my best visits occur when I bring something with me. Interest is sparked and a topic of discussion is obvious from the beginning. There is a flow. Time doesn't seem to drag.

Consider this: Many family members find that bringing their relative favorite food items sparks reminiscent conversation. Cherry phosphates, chocolate malts, or a carefully prepared old family recipe can be excellent stimuli for creating happy exchanges. One family brings apples to an elderly relative who had owned and operated an apple orchard. In the facility's kitchen they prepare applesauce, pies, and jelly together.

Sharing the Care

Getting along with others was never a problem for my loved one. In fact, it's important to her to be pleasant and amiable. She has always been well liked and had lots of friends.

Consider this: Some residents will never "rock a boat" themselves. If they are upset about the way something is done in the facility or have a problem with certain members of the staff, they seldom complain directly. Their family members are the ones who hear all their complaints. This makes it hard on the family because the elderly loved one desires to appear friendly and nice to everyone else. She wants to be liked. The family must face the issues themselves. Sometimes this can be done successfully through the local ombudsman.

Sharing the Care

Environmental changes can greatly help or control actions, which might otherwise be viewed as bad or unmanageable behavior. Adjusting the environment or creating activities to discourage unacceptable behavior can often make a world of difference. There must be a proper fit between a person and his environment.

Consider this: Some facilities have provisions for residents who are awake a lot during the night. This is especially helpful for Alzheimer's patients who may have sleep reversal or experience sundowning. A safe, well-lit area is provided. An activity is usually going on and the room is manned by a staff member. The space might be called a launderers' lounge where the residents help fold the clean laundry.

Sharing the Care

I realize that most of the personal attention and care my loved one receives is from me and the aides. I believe I am the one most apt to pursue what I perceive as a health problem. Whenever I observe something that concerns me, I ask the nurse in charge to look at it as soon as possible.

Consider this: Most long-term care facilities make arrangements for regularly scheduled visits by specialty health care professionals. Dentists, podiatrists, and ophthalmologists are among the many who may be needed. Be aware of these visits and let the staff know when you feel your relative requires special attention. You might want to periodically check your relative's feet for ingrown or extremely long toenails. Bad breath or wincing when chewing could indicate a dental problem.

Sharing the Care

   Mealtime is an important time for all of us. It takes on even greater significance if the rest of our day isn't very busy. I understand why the quality of the meals and the atmosphere of the dining room are crucial elements in my loved one's life.

Consider this: The biggest social event in your relative's day may very well be mealtime. If you haven't stayed for a meal with him, try to do so. Or, at least arrange to end a visit right before dinner and accompany him to the dining room before you leave. Observe the food and how it is prepared and presented. Notice the seating arrangements. Ask if they change places periodically to encourage sociability. Be aware of whether your relative looks forward to meals or not. If not, find out why.

Sharing the Care

Most of the residents of the care facility love to have a good time. I'm always on the outlook for new and creative ways to help them enjoy life and add quality to their days.

Consider this: One facility's family council presented a unique program for the residents. They put together a style show with family members wearing vintage clothing. The music they played was appropriate to the era of the apparel worn by each model. Items such as unlit oil lamps, mantel clocks, and old dolls were carried by the models. Antique jewelry, pocket watches and fobs were worn. An old-fashioned ice cream social rounded out the afternoon. Family members, staff, and residents mingled and admired all the memorabilia!

Sharing the Care

People don't seem to dance like they used to. How long has it been since I heard someone say they were going out dancing? What has happened to this wonderful form of entertainment? Maybe we're missing something today. Let's go dancing!

Consider this: Dancing is a wonderful activity for the residents of care facilities. It is generally safe and can be enjoyed by all. Lots of residents "dance" while seated in their wheel chairs. Dementia patients usually love to join in. It is non-threatening, encourages exercise, and uses up excess energy. Old familiar tunes, especially ones from the Big Band era are great hits with most residents.

Sharing the Care

Some people are more easily annoyed than others. We all have different tolerance levels. I try to understand when something just isn't acceptable to my loved one.

Consider this: Occasionally, roommates will get on each other's nerves—or worse. Some residents require a great deal of privacy. If one roommate wants to listen to music and the other does not or one plays the radio too loud, personal headsets may be in order. Color-coding their belongings often works if items get borrowed without permission. Personality conflicts can be a factor at any age. If your best efforts to encourage compatibility fail, a room transfer for your relative may be necessary.

Sharing the Care

Unlike animals, people are not just "body-conscious." Human beings definitely have a spiritual side. Some of us are more in touch with it than others. This element of our make-up enables us to reflect on our lives and recognize the blessings we've enjoyed.

Consider this: If your relative has a strong spiritual sense, allow him to express his reflections of life as a whole. It's healthy for him to look at the happenings of his life and to have an acceptance of them and of the people who have touched him along the way.

Sharing the Care

So many things have changed in my loved one's lifetime! Technology seems to be racing past him at a pace he can't keep up with or even imagine. Sometimes I long for a quieter, simpler time too.

Consider this: Be careful not to antiquate or put down ideas dear to your elderly relative. Don't dismiss his views. Listen to him and learn from him. Perhaps, you'll benefit from a strictly historical advantage— or maybe you'll begin to see how his views could help the future. They may even go hand-in-hand with today's ideas to form an even better world tomorrow.

Sharing the Care

At times I feel guilty for not taking care of my loved one at home. Those are the times I must make a reality check. I observe the care he is getting in the facility. I see how many aides it takes to lift him, to change his garments—to provide the amount of care he now requires. I must periodically face the fact I could not adequately care for him at home. It may sadden me, but there is no reason for me to feel guilty. I can replace sadness with the joy of knowing he is being cared for by many capable people.

Consider this: Frequent reality checks on your part will also make you aware of any unnecessary assistance you or the staff provides your relative. He should be encouraged and allowed to do as much for himself as he is able.

Sharing the Care

What my loved one sees in my eyes and in my manner, may very well be the picture she sees of herself. Do I look at her with love, or reproach? Do I treat her with respect, or disdain? What does she hear in my tone of voice? Am I condescending, or do I talk to her as an equal?

Consider this: The role of the ill and the elderly in our culture is rather undefined. Ours is such a productivity-oriented society. When someone is no longer able to produce an income they are apt to consider themselves less worthy—because unfortunately that's the unspoken message that is often implied. We, as loving family members must assure our ill or elderly relatives they will always be valued.

Sharing the Care

My loved one and his friends at the facility need to feel useful. Most of them can do a lot more than they are currently doing. They just need encouragement and some fresh ideas once in a while.

Consider this: Consider getting together with family members of other residents and suggesting to the residents some worthwhile project they could do together for their community. It can foster pride, camaraderie, and the good feeling that comes from helping others. It will provide something to look forward to and increase their sense of self-worth. Keeping ties with the community and life outside the care facility whenever possible is stimulating and healthy.

Sharing the Care

Life should be a process of continuous growth from birth till death. Aging and retirement need not mean retiring from living and learning. My loved one has a future and a present, as well as a past. She may have stopped doing some things, but she certainly can still continue to develop herself in other ways.

Consider this: Long-term care facilities should have adequate libraries for their residents. If yours does not, ask if you can help create one or improve the existing one. Make sure it includes not only the classics, but books with new ideas and concepts. Don't forget audiocassettes, books in large print, and Braille if needed. Provide plenty of large picture books for residents with Alzheimer's disease. Residents need to know about the library and its contents.

Sharing the Care

When I visit my loved one, I sit down near him. If there isn't a chair there, I get one. I'm not comfortable standing if he is seated or lying down. I don't want to appear big and powerful or in any way cause him to feel small or insignificant. I sit close to him at his level so I can look into his eyes and give him my full attention and the respect he deserves.

Consider this: Ask your relative if he is having any difficulties functioning in his surroundings. His room should have adequate storage for his clothing and other personal items. Check to make sure the light switches in his room and bathroom are easy for him to locate and reach. His towel bars should be installed at a good level for him.

Sharing the Care

Not only is it important for my loved one to be cared for, I believe it is important for her to be able to give care, too. There are still opportunities for her to show care for others—family members, fellow residents, and members of the community.

Consider this: Many churches recognize the prayer potential that exists among the elderly. They often share their prayer lists with care facility residents who know how to pray for the specific needs of others. Also if your relative can do mending, set tables in the facility, read stories to visiting children, or push her roommate's wheelchair—she will seldom feel lonely or bored. Ministering to someone else's needs almost always cures loneliness and self-pity. Facilities are finding that even caring for small pets does wonders for their residents.

Sharing the Care

     Why do men usually act like they don't want any fuss made over them? Do they really mean it? I still try to make a big deal out of special occasions like Father's Day. He can object all he wants to, but our family is going to celebrate him!

Consider this: Father's Day festivities are fun to plan, partly because of the time of year. Most men enjoy being outdoors. Outings to a special fishing lake in the community or a picnic on the facility grounds make for a memorable day. Some facilities plan a special sports day inside or outside. Indoor activities might include viewing sports videos—or perhaps consider scheduling an appearance by the coach or players of a local high school, college, or professional sports team.

Sharing the Care

My loved one's safety is of extreme importance to me. I trust she is cared for as protectively as possible without taking her rights away. I want her to feel comfortable and secure, but not limited unnecessarily in her privileges.

Consider this: All elements of your relative's well being should be addressed by the care facility. If you feel they are lacking in some area, discuss it with them in a non-threatening manner. Many facilities require all visitors to sign in when they enter and to sign out upon leaving. Deliveries are left with the receptionist. Knowledge of a code number is needed to enter and to leave secure units.

Sharing the Care

I let my loved one know he has an impact on future generations—the younger members of our own family in particular. It's important for the old and young to spend some time together. Even if the elderly member is only able to hold the youngest member on his lap, a connection is formed.

Consider this: People of like age may find themselves grouped together in school settings, social functions, and in long-term care facilities, but age segregation is not a good idea. Inter-generational activities and cross-generational sharing is essential for a healthy society. All ages seem to benefit by coexisting—and sometimes just by quietly observing each other.

Sharing the Care

I urge everyone who has been a part of my loved one's life to remain in contact with her. Friends, former neighbors, former in-home-care helpers, all have a standing invitation to visit her. Sometimes I plan a get-together in the party room and send out invitations.

Consider this: Maintaining friendships and relationships is as meaningful as making new ones. Physical surroundings shouldn't affect the interaction between people, but sometimes they do. Some people will need a little nudge or a special invitation before they feel welcome or comfortable visiting your relative in the new environment.

Sharing the Care

Change can be difficult at any age. My loved one has weathered many changes in her lifetime. Nevertheless, some changes today seem difficult for her.

Consider this: Changes in the environment or even changes in staff shifts can have an effect on the residents, especially those experiencing dementia. Any change in a comfortable and familiar atmosphere can be the cause of difficult behavior, frustration, or sadness among some individuals. Many care facilities plan a special group activity for each shift change. A non-threatening pastime such as a sing-a-long can take the attention away from the bustling numbers of staff coming and going—and replace the momentary awareness of missing a favorite staff member who is going off duty.

Sharing the Care

Some things in life just seem to elicit joy. Sunshine, a child's natural laughter, kites, and beach balls come to mind. They are all freeing! When I am with my loved one I try to introduce joyful activities and memories. They usually relieve him of any heaviness he is feeling.

Consider this: Puppets can spread joy and bring lightness into most situations. Their appeal generally has no age limits. Try introducing a puppet or two into your relative's life. He may enjoy having one of his own. A group of residents might want to become puppeteers and create entertaining shows for guests of all ages, fellow residents—or even other care facilities!

Sharing the Care

The quality of my loved one's environment is extremely important. The emotional atmosphere is as much a part of the environment as the physical aspects. A friendly, safe, and relaxed setting means more to our family than fancy or trendy interior decorating.

Consider this: The activity room should be comfortable and inviting—like a warm kitchen or cozy family room. It's a gathering place where cookies can be baking, a jigsaw puzzle might be in progress, or a craft is being worked on. Modernized facilities are placing ovens at the eye level of those seated in wheelchairs. For the safety of dementia residents, ovens can be closed behind cabinet doors when not in use and stove tops installed with flip-top counter tops like those used in campers.

Sharing the Care

We all age from the day we are born. Sometimes my loved one and I discuss what we call successful aging. We take an inventory of where we both are in our lives. We both want to continue to absorb new things every day. We talk about the things we're learning and what we're doing with this knowledge.

Consider this: Every day can be filled with new things and be a learning experience no matter what our age or environment. Motivate your relative to continue to take things in and to continue to learn. There might be something he has always wanted to study, but never had the time before. There are many books, audiocassettes, videos, and correspondence courses he could take advantage of no matter what his age or limited physical abilities.

Sharing the Care

My loved one may require care in some ways, but she can still function on her own at full capacity in other ways. I refuse to let her or anyone else dwell on what she cannot do. It's much healthier to focus on what she can do and what she still does well. Stressing the positives in life has always made more sense to me than getting bogged down on the negatives.

Consider this: Many care facility residents who cannot walk, might need help with some activities of daily living, but can still do most activities independently and should be encouraged to do so.

Sharing the Care

Safety is a major consideration in the administration of a care facility. It's a big enough responsibility for most families in an average size house. I appreciate the precautions the staff has to take in a large congregate living setting. From the care of the floors to the cleanliness of the kitchen, it's an awesome responsibility.

Consider this: Inquire whether your relative's home engages in fire drills. Is there adequate staff to evacuate everyone quickly—especially at night? Can they do it calmly? Are all members of the staff well trained for emergencies?

Sharing the Care

Privacy is something everyone is entitled to. I respect my loved one's privacy. Her physical privacy and her mental privacy. I realize her thoughts are private, too. She may not want to share all of them with me. That's okay.

Consider this: Everyone—family and staff—should knock before entering a resident's room. Unfortunately, not all residents respect the privacy of fellow residents. Confused residents often disturb others without intending to do so. Nevertheless, it is upsetting to those whose privacy they are intruding upon. Some facilities do not integrate confused or dementia residents with cognitive residents. They reside in a separate area of the facility.

Sharing the Care

I realize the activity director is much more than an entertainment organizer. She actually cares about my relative's interests, experiences, abilities, and well being. She knows him as well as any other staff member does, maybe even better. I appreciate the caring way she does her job.

Consider this: The sound of music playing or the smell of something baking can bring someone out of their room more effectively than any amount of coaxing ever could. Staff members cannot force anyone to join in activities. Residents have the right to decide for themselves what they do and don't do. They are adults and are free to fill their time with whatever they choose, but innovative and creative staff can successfully entice the most stubborn residents—sometimes with inviting sounds and aromas.

Sharing the Care

My loved one has developed a definite sense of belonging in the care facility. She seems to feel secure and protected in the environment.

Consider this: Many residents feel very safe once they have adjusted to living in a long-term care facility. Some have moved from neighborhoods they had begun to view as unsafe. They read of violence in the world outside. Now that their world has grown smaller and more predictable, they feel secure and protected among the walls of the facility.

Sharing the Care

The care of my loved one is enhanced when it is a sharing process. The staff, our family, and when possible, our relative herself, all contribute to her care and the quality of her life in the facility. We exchange ideas, observations, and concerns.

Consider this: The family should always be a part of any decision-making process involving a change that personally affects their relative. Families and residents do better with recommendations rather than being told by the staff that a decision has been made regarding a change in a care procedure, a medical treatment, or a level of care. Everyone needs to be well-informed regarding residents' rights, medical directives, and health care proxies.

Sharing the Care

Common interests bring people together. Sharing similar experiences, performing like tasks, and possessing mutual beliefs or concerns can form bonds in people who don't necessarily have a history together.

Consider this: We all grew up knowing the value of community spirit. Whether the community is a school, a town, a church or synagogue, belonging and working together for common goals is healthy. The residents, family members, and staff share a common bond and interest—the facility itself. Pride in it and working together to make it the best it can be promotes a wonderful bond and a mutual interest.

Sharing the Care

Caring for plants is a pleasant and emotionally healthy experience. Plants are not only nice to look at—they need us! They require lots of loving care only we can give them.

Consider this: A garden room with sunny windows, special lighting, sinks, cabinets, and ample working space is a pleasant addition to any home. Care facilities find that such a room delights residents, provides another interest, is an alternative gathering place, and it gives many residents something to look forward to every day. Consider starting a garden club in your facility. Local garden clubs might like to be involved in sponsoring programs for the residents.

Sharing the Care

Children are generally accepting and loving. Kids just seem to look beyond some of the stuff we adults get hung up on. Their views and reactions to the world around them are inspiring. We all need children in our lives once in a while to remind us of those qualities and help restore them in us!

Consider this: Children provide a connection with the good in life. They are spontaneous and remind us not to take life or ourselves too seriously. Scouts, 4-H clubs, and church youth groups form lasting bonds with the elderly when they combine projects and programs with long-term care facilities. Suggest such a connection with a youth organization you are familiar with.

Sharing the Care

I feel refreshed after a good laugh. The responsibilities of caregiving, the stress of everyday life, and trying to juggle numerous duties often leaves me burdened and with little humor. Some days I fail to see anything funny in my life. So, I've decided to pursue some form of comedy at least once a day.

Consider this: All of us can benefit from a good healthy laugh. Try reading something funny, listening to comedy tapes, and viewing comedy movies. Some family members bring joke or gag items to the facility when they visit. Wearing tastefully humorous T-shirts or buttons can elicit smiles. One visitor goes through his relative's entire facility once a week with a "humor cart."

Sharing the Care

I'm thankful for a care facility that promotes social interaction between residents, staff, and family members. The bonds being formed not only help to better the cooperation between us, they make our facility a friendly and enjoyable place to live, work, and visit.

Consider this: A baby picture party is a good ice-breaking get-together. Try to obtain a baby picture from all who plan to attend. At the party, exhibit a large poster with everyone's baby picture on it and number each picture, but don't put their names by the pictures. Have everyone wear a nametag and give everyone a pencil and paper. Attendees talk, mingle, and get better acquainted by trying to see how many people they can match with their pictures. Some groups have prizes for those with the most correct, followed by a potluck dinner or snacks.

Sharing the Care

I hope my loved one is comfortable and at peace with his surroundings and with his family. I know having familiar things and people around him contributes greatly to his comfort level.

Consider this: Sometimes we are uncomfortable with the unfamiliar. Some people flee when they are frustrated, fearful, or uncomfortable. Often, if someone cannot flee physically, they flee inwardly. If your relative seems to be withdrawing, try to determine what he might be fearful of, or uncomfortable with. Is something frustrating him? Talk with other family members and the staff to see what can be done to increase his comfort level.

Sharing the Care

As with all of us, it's important for my loved one to be comfortable with who she is. She has no problem asserting herself and letting her desires be known. I'm proud of her self-assurance and I tell her so!

Consider this: Most elderly people have learned to do what works. They've reached a time in life when they want sensible and comfortable clothing. Fashion is not an issue. They no longer feel a need to compete. They don't yield to a pressure to conform. We can certainly learn something from them!

Sharing the Care

Nature is uplifting. Whenever the weather permits, I try to take my loved one outside. The environment is good for both of us. The garden area of the facility provides welcome sunshine, plants, wild birds, and an occasional squirrel or two for our enjoyment and pleasure.

Consider this: Large indoor fish tanks and even indoor birdcages and aviaries delight residents and visitors in many facilities today. They provide entertainment and spontaneity. Something new and different is always happening in them. Some residents enjoy helping care for the fish and birds.

Sharing the Care

People need to be able to make choices. Without choices we feel we have lost control. I'm conscious of giving my loved one as many choices in his life as possible. Circumstances beyond our control have made some choices impossible. So, I look for ways he can be in control and be given some choices of his own.

Consider this: Most elderly people have experienced many losses. The loss of control over some of the circumstances in one's life is just part of life. But, being able to make choices is needed for everyone's self-esteem. Dementia patients can be confused by too many choices, however being offered simple choices between one shirt or another, or one type of beverage over another is important.

Sharing the Care

I try to see the care facility as a big family. When I do so, I am more understanding of their problems. Many people in the family are ill and have special needs. The facility is on a budget just like any other family. There are meals to prepare, rooms to clean, laundry to do, and grounds to maintain. Personalities and moods need to be dealt with. I believe the facility functions pretty well as a family.

Consider this: Some care facilities encourage family members of their residents to form a family council. Some also have resident councils. The councils, the staff, and the local ombudsman all work together for the betterment of the facility and the care of its residents.

Sharing the Care

Our family takes advantage of our relative's years of experience. He has plenty of time now to pass his knowledge and wisdom on to us. He is a veteran of life. All the members of our family learn from him.

Consider this: The elderly can help pass on valued traditions—especially to the youth in their families. They might help prepare the younger members of the family for bar mitzvahs, bat mitzvahs, confirmations, scout badges, and so on. There are many wonderful ways they can assist today's busy parents and help assure the direction the children and teens are guided in. Learn to use this rich and valuable resource. Doing so will also validate a sense of usefulness and purposefulness in your elderly relative.

Sharing the Care

I try to take my time when I'm with my loved one. It's actually good for me to slow my normal pace. I usually feel refreshed and less harassed after a visit with her. Her world is not as complicated as mine. Sometimes I'm envious!

Consider this: If you take your relative for an outing outside the care facility, be prepared to allow plenty of time. Hurrying will frustrate both of you. Extra time will certainly be needed if a wheelchair is involved, but even if your relative walks, she is probably not used to walking at your pace. Adjust to hers. Plan any excursion as a celebration and enjoy the special time together.

Sharing the Care

Mealtime is always a special time in our family. I'm so glad the care facility recognizes it as special, too. My loved one looks forward to dining with his friends every day. The atmosphere is always clean, friendly, and cheerful.

Consider this: Not all care facilities use meal trays. In fact, more and more of them are finding advantages to serving family-style meals. The atmosphere is more home-like and comfortable. Some facilities offer restaurant-style dining with table servers. In both the family-style approach and the restaurant atmosphere, table linens and china are used—rather than individual trays.

Sharing the Care

During difficult times I am especially thankful for the extended family I have through the care facility. The loving consideration of the staff, the residents, and other families makes such a difference when we struggle through a crisis together.

Consider this: When a resident is seriously ill or dying, the needs of family members and roommates must be met—along with those of the patient. Often a cot will be provided for a close family member to stay overnight, if they so desire. During this time, arrangements are often made for the roommate to temporarily move to another room. One of the rooms set aside for respite use might be used for this purpose.

Sharing the Care

Working together on a project gives the residents something to look forward to every day. It also helps to keep the group cohesive. In fact, the results are usually so positive, they begin a new project just as soon as one is completed!

Consider this: In one facility the residents got together and created a cookbook. The contributions were from both women and men. They had it printed and sold copies in their local hospital gift shop and other shops in the community. The recipes were wonderful! The volume also contained interesting stories and old traditions. The proceeds went to the residents' council. They used the funds for many useful items and good causes.

Sharing the Care

The residents and the staff members appear to know each other well. They even seem to understand when someone is having a bad day. They support one another like family.

Consider this: Some facilities find one way to insure a close bond between the staff and the residents is to have a different member of the staff be a guest at each residents' council meeting. Staff members tell a little about themselves, their family, and what their job entails. The residents can ask questions and get to know each staff person individually in a mutually relaxing atmosphere.

Sharing the Care

I'm working on keeping everything in the proper perspective. I don't smother my loved one. Conversely, I don't dismiss her either. I believe we have a good adult relationship. I don't resent the attention she requires. The time I spend with her and on her care is reasonable and acceptable to me.

Consider this: The most successful family caregivers are the ones who are honest with themselves and their loved ones. They are realistic about the time they give to caregiving. They realize if they feel pushed or over-obligated, they will harbor resentments. They generally feel comfortable and accepting of the situation and the circumstances. They take good care of themselves, as well as their care recipients.

Sharing the Care

Sometimes the elderly themselves exhibit a negative view of aging. I discourage my loved one from any such degrading stereotypes. It hurts to hear him put himself and his age group down. I tell him we need their wisdom, strength, and guidance. A society that focuses only on youth won't be very successful in the long run.

Consider this: Unfortunately, self-esteem among the elderly is often very fragile. They need to believe in themselves. Look for ways to uplift and reassure your relative of his value to you, your family, and society as a whole. Where would we be without him and his peers? Let him know he is valued.

Sharing the Care

I'm amazed and thrilled at the amount of interest most of the residents take in the facility and in each other. It's a joy to see them so involved in life. They help make the facility the successful community it is.

Consider this: When encouraged and allowed to, residents can be the best volunteers a facility has. Many residents organize and run facility gift shops. Some even provide a cart service making daily rounds to fellow residents who are unable to get to the gift shop or the facility's library. Residents often want to care for the gardens and courtyard grounds. The number of areas residents can volunteer their help is inexhaustible!

Sharing the Care

Our society doesn't discuss aging very well—or very often. I'd like to be able to talk about it and learn more about it. I want to help my aging loved one with any struggles he may be having. Being knowledgeable and comfortable with the subject of aging will also help me as I continue to age.

Consider this: Communication breaks down misconceptions and misunderstandings. Ask elders questions about aging. Encourage them to talk about their image of aging. Is their image different from what they feel it should be? Discuss how our culture's attitude toward the aging process and its elders can improve.

Sharing the Care

My loved one needs to be in a professional care facility for the degree of care she now requires. In this congregate setting, we do everything we can to prevent her from experiencing feelings of depersonalization. Her room contains all the special things that personalize it for her. The staff members address her by name and treat her with attentive care and consideration.

Consider this: No one wants to be treated like a non-person. Being treated like just another number among many residents under a common roof is terribly upsetting. Listen to the way the staff talks to your relative. Observe the overall way they treat people. If you or your relative feel there is a problem, speak to the facility administration. If the situation does not improve, you may want to seek another facility.

Sharing the Care

Helping someone and making a positive difference in their life makes us feel better about ourselves. It also provides us with an interest apart from our own problems. Reaching out to another person is always a good idea!

Consider this: Your relative might enjoy sponsoring a child in another country. There are many agencies to consider. For a small monthly contribution he can help feed and clothe a child in a less fortunate part of the world. A photo of the child is usually sent to the sponsor. Correspondence is encouraged. You and other members of your family may wish to provide the monthly contribution if the financial participation is a problem for your loved one.

Sharing the Care

We can learn a lot about patriotism from those who have lived longer than us. Sometimes we forget how fortunate we are. We may need to be reminded. Other generations sacrificed for the freedoms we enjoy and often take for granted.

Consider this: Elderly countrymen can pass along to younger generations a great heritage and pride in our country. Many facilities bring area school children together with the residents on legal holidays. The children might hear patriotic stories they haven't heard from their parents. History books can come alive!

Sharing the Care

The spontaneity of animals provides something many facilities overlook. My loved one has always enjoyed having a pet of her own. Why should that stop now? Today more than ever she needs all the companionship and interests available to her.

Consider this: Many long-term care facilities are allowing and providing the opportunity for residents to have parakeets or finches in their rooms. Some residents care for the cages themselves. Often staff members share the responsibilities. In some homes family members keep the cages clean and provide the bird food. Occasionally residents enjoy having a gold fish or Betta fish in a bowl. A personal pet is a comfort and can relieve boredom and loneliness.

Sharing the Care

I appreciate everything the facility does to make my loved one's life enjoyable and of the best quality. Whatever they can do to play down the feeling of being an institution helps immensely in the overall well being of the residents.

Consider this: Depending on the staff and the circumstances, meals served on individual trays may be the only answer for some facilities. But, when possible meals presented and served family-style provide a much more enjoyable and familiar atmosphere in which to eat. Facilities that are able to accomplish a home-like environment for meals are providing an important element in the comfort and care level of its residents.

Sharing the Care

Having a common goal and purpose gives meaning to our lives and promotes community enthusiasm and pride. The residents of the facility brighten up when they are working together on something.

Consider this: An active residents' council may want to open a resident-operated gift shop for residents and visitors. Small gifts, cards, stationery, artwork, craft items, and candies can be among the merchandise offered. Some of the items might even be produced by the residents themselves.

Sharing the Care

There is no excuse for boredom in our facility. When family members and activity staff take the time to suggest ideas and provide areas for residents to pursue varied interests, creativity flourishes. The results are delightful for everyone involved.

Consider this: Growing fragrant herbs and flowers can be a satisfying activity in itself. Drying them and creating floral arrangements, or putting herbs into attractive jars for kitchen use provide hours of activity and creativity. Marketable gift items and lovely decorations are another by-product. All ages take pride in growing things and in making useful and beautiful gifts.

Sharing the Care

Having fun shouldn't cease just because of advanced age or health limitations. Opportunities for socialization and companionship in the facility should not be any different from the community in general. The possibilities are limitless if we'll just use our imaginations.

Consider this: One innovative facility turned a cozy room into a "men's only" sports bar. Sports posters and lighted signs hang on the walls. A pool table, poker tables, and game machines provide hours of fun. Weekly card games are very popular. The facility provides pretzels, peanuts, and non-alcoholic beer. The residents have even formed teams. The teams challenge each other on the game machines and in pool tournaments.

Sharing the Care

People who are already familiar and comfortable with long term-care facilities have an easier time making decisions and adjustments when this level of care is needed for a loved one. There are many ways people can become involved in a care facility in their community.

Consider this: Priests, rabbis, and ministers shouldn't be the only members of their congregations who make visits to local care facilities. Some have members who regularly volunteer and help out in any way they can in this outreach. Youth groups have a wonderful opportunity of on-going ministry and sharing in care facilities. There is much more that can be done in this area than just showing up during the holidays and singing carols.

Sharing the Care

Everyone has distinct tastes and preferences. These choices make us who we are and help define our individual uniqueness. Whenever my loved one has the opportunity to make choices of his own and retain his special identity, he does so.

Consider this: Residents' rooms should evidence their personalities and individualities. Favorite craft items and hobbies of the past or present can be displayed. Meaningful pictures and photos of special times and events should be prominent. Don't forget to include awards and trophies. If the facility allows, selection of individual bedspreads and window treatments for each person's room provides further personal expression.

Sharing the Care

Small pleasures and good care go hand-in-hand. Ministering to someone's physical and emotional needs are often easy to combine. I am thankful for a care facility that understands and looks for ways to fill my loved one's needs.

Consider this: Afternoon snack carts can provide a refreshing break and a special time to look forward to. A cheerful volunteer or aide offering choices of soda, juices, fruits, and home-made desserts or cookies is a welcome addition to anyone's day. A feeling of loving care and friendliness can be conveyed at the same time needed liquids and nutritional snacks are added to the day's diet.

Sharing the Care

Separation implies being apart from someone. My loved one and I may not live together, but nothing can really separate us emotionally. The physical separation is something we cannot control. One squeeze of the hand or a reassuring hug affirms the connection we will always have.

Consider this: People suffering from dementia often retain adequate social skills. They usually enjoy exchanging pleasant greetings and engaging in short, light conversations. The emotional well being of all participants can be enhanced by these exchanges.

Sharing the Care

We're stimulated by the sights and sounds of life around us. When spontaneous things happen, conversation and interest often flourish.

Consider this: Many care facilities are intentionally built adjacent to parks, school yards, and sports fields. Their residents always have something to watch through windows and outdoor access. Wonderful sounds can be heard. Children playing, bands practicing, football games, and outdoor concerts all provide hours of varied stimulus and pleasure.

Sharing the Care

An atmosphere of "homeness" is most important for my loved one. The personalities of care facilities can be as varied as our individual homes. We sought a facility that most resembled our home.

Consider this: Sunny windows with sills for plants, good pleasant aromas, friendly pets, toys and some furniture for visiting children, cozy places to sit, and outdoor gardens can all be found in many of today's long-term care facilities. Know what is important to your relative and your family. Try not to settle for less!

Sharing the Care

My loved one doesn't have much chance to be bored. He is encouraged to be involved in a number of activities offered by the facility and our family. Life does not stop just because he changed his address!

Consider this: Many facilities offer two or three outings a week for residents who are able to be transported in the facility vehicles. Trips to malls, outdoor markets, local libraries, restaurants, special exhibits, and other points of interest should be available to all who can participate.

Sharing the Care

My loved one was raised with a strong work ethic. Now that he is no longer active in the working force, he often acts like he doesn't feel good about himself. He says his skills are outmoded. He is apologetic about not working. I tell him I understand, but he is much more than the work he did. I reassure him of his continuing value to society and to our family. I remind him of the wonderful contributions he is still making to us.

Consider this: Quite often elderly people equate their worth with previous occupations. If they are no longer able to perform their vocations, they may feel useless. Our society needs to do all we can to let them know it is they themselves who are important to us.

Sharing the Care

I'm happy to see our community taking a greater interest and pride in its long-term care facilities. I will do everything I can to encourage a bond between the community and the facility administration for the betterment of the residents.

Consider this: Many long-term care facilities have adopted the name "Living Center"—realizing life and involvement with the community don't get checked in at the door. Child and adult day care facilities are often located on the same campuses as long-term care facilities. Interaction between all the generations is fostered and incorporated into everyone's daily life.

Sharing the Care

I am grateful for my loved one. She is the one person in my world who sits still and really listens to me. She hears my words. When I ask her for direction, she sifts my problems through the sands of time, wisdom, and experience. When she gives her advice, I know she has considered things I have not thought of. I listen to her and know she will not judge me—no matter what I do.

Consider this: The bond between two people of different generations can be a special blessing to both. Each brings different things to the table. What a celebration of life!

Sharing the Care

Labeling people does grave injustice to individuals. No two old people are alike No two young people are alike. Everyone with dementia does not behave the same. We must avoid labels. They prohibit us from seeing the person behind the tag we've so hastily and thoughtlessly placed on them. There is no room for labels in a truly loving environment.

Consider this: Successful staff and family members can see past outer problems to the hearts of people. Age, physical handicaps, or dementia don't change what's inside a person. Recognizing and treating someone's inner spirit must come first in all forms of human care.

Sharing the Care

I look for unique and meaningful gifts to give my loved one. Practical things are fine and often needed, but I am delighted when I can get him something he'll really enjoy.

Consider this: Old photos can be put on video. Someone whose eyesight is dimming may be able to view them better on a large television screen rather than in a photo album. One lady spends hours watching videos of old photos her family had made for her. Appropriate and meaningful background music can be an added feature to the videos and provides even more enjoyment.

Sharing the Care

When I see my loved one sitting with her hands folded motionless on her lap, I wonder if it is a sign of composure and contentment—or are they folded inward? Do her idle hands long to be busy again? To reach out to others?

Consider this: When we're involved with life, our hands just seem to move. Whether we're telling a story, sharing an idea, shelling peas, or petting a dog, our hands become a vital and animated part of life. You might get idle hands involved again by asking your relative to help you with something.

Sharing the Care

By keeping our eyes, ears, and hearts open, we find there are many opportunities to add joy and spontaneity to the care facility.

Consider this: A group of gentlemen residents were reminiscing about electric train sets they enjoyed when they were younger. Some family members and staff got wind of this interest. They set aside an area large enough for a wheelchair-accessible platform. Together, interested staff, family members, and residents collected and repaired old train sets. They built a miniature village with adaptations for changes in seasons. This welcome addition provides many happy hours for everyone. Visiting children are drawn to it and residents love showing it off to the younger set.

Sharing the Care

My loved one has tastes and habits that needn't be discouraged. Retaining them preserves her dignity and her right to make choices for herself. If she is comfortable with something or doing something and it doesn't threaten her safety or the safety of others, we let her do it.

Consider this: Aprons can still be very practical and popular. They are fresh and perky. Their pockets hold any number of things. Cobbler aprons protect clothing when eating. Aprons can have a familiarity to former homemakers and are more adult and dignified than bibs. If large bibs are used for adults, get into the habit of calling them "fabric protectors"—not bibs!

Sharing the Care

My loved one really has no need for cash now. However, he insists on having some with him. It's a security issue for him. So, I make sure he has a few dollars in his wallet and some change in his pocket—an amount small enough that it won't be a problem if it is lost or given away.

Consider this: If your relative has Alzheimer's disease or a related disorder, artificial paper money or plastic cards that look like credit cards may be appropriate for him to carry. When dementia patients ask to have money, sometimes they are satisfied if you tell them their money is safe in the bank where you are watching it for them.

Sharing the Care

I try to put myself in someone else's place. When I am able to understand what they experience and what they see from their perspective, I am better able to meet their needs effectively.

Consider this: People naturally see things like signs, mirrors, directions, wall hangings and calendars when they are mounted at eye-level. In a care facility, there are two eye-levels to be considered—one from a standing position and the other from the seat of a wheelchair.

Sharing the Care

Wherever I look, I see wonderful ingredients and ideas for activities. They abound in the everyday life that surrounds me. All I have to do is use my senses and my imagination.

Consider this: Taste and smell are wonderful sensory stimulants. Kitchens hold exquisite keys that unlock secret memories. It is a storehouse of materials that can open doors to marvelous reminiscence and discussions. Mint, wintergreen, vanilla, and almond—the kitchen is full of them!

Sharing the Care

Taking time often saves time. It can relieve anxieties on everyone's part. A slower, more thoughtful pace eases stress and often discourages troublesome behaviors. When we take the time, we can usually avoid problems.

Consider this: Vision-impaired residents and residents with dementia often have difficulty walking over different floor textures. When walking with them, take your time. Gently take their arm. Explain the change in flooring. It may help to stop and have them look at or feel the floor before stepping on it. This is especially helpful when moving from a hard floor onto carpet.

Sharing the Care

Boundaries are important at any age. They need to be respected and preserved. I don't ever want my loved one to feel his personal boundaries are open for anyone to step all over.

Consider this: The way voice and touch are used has a definite impact on the emotional security of those they are directed toward. Loud voices and rough touch are abusive. No one should be approached suddenly from behind. If someone is being moved, they should be told first—in a loving manner. Moving someone in their wheelchair without explaining why or where they are being taken makes them feel helpless and unimportant.

Sharing the Care

Exercising positive free expression is part of being in control of your life. Doing something for the fun of it can add a spark to your day and brighten the lives of others.

Consider this: Try leaving any fun accessories you can think of like hats, wigs, or old sunglasses in the activity room. Watch the joy and freedom of expression it provides both staff and residents as they pick them up and put them on. It can break monotony, encourage laughter, and discourage boredom.

Sharing the Care

Doing harmless silly things as a group brings people closer. Coming together on a nonsensical level puts everyone at ease. Moods are lifted and the endorphins rule.

Consider this: Some schools and offices have casual and dress-up days. Going a step farther, one care facility declared Saturdays as T-shirt or sweatshirt days. Self-expression and whimsy flourish for both residents and staff. Regular visitors even get in on the act!

Sharing the Care

We all need ways of exercising our independence. Making choices during the day, whether big or small, allows us to be individuals. I realize this is as important for my loved one as is it for me.

Consider this: Congregate living tends to breed conformity, rather than individuality. Dependent persons need to find sources of self-expression and satisfaction. Activity directors and concerned family members must be aware of this need. Residents should be allowed to make a number of decisions for themselves, within the realm of safety and within their capabilities. A certain amount of flexibility can be achieved in the congregate setting. Some suggestions may be offering menu selections, flexible mealtimes, and choices between numerous and varied daily activities.

Sharing the Care

My loved one's opportunities to show affection are more limited now. She has always been loving and given so much love to our family. I wish I could spend more time with her, but my job and responsibilities outside the care facility take up a great deal of my time.

Consider this: Many Alzheimer's patients seem to derive satisfaction from holding, talking to, petting, and showing affection to stuffed animals. Baby dolls are also very popular and appear to fill a void and a need. If your relative finds comfort in a stuffed animal or doll, don't be embarrassed and don't discourage the attachment.

Sharing the Care

Punishment is not appropriate for adults whose behavior may be deemed inappropriate. Grown-ups resent being scolded or threatened for doing something someone in authority disapproves of.

Consider this: Residents with dementia may become agitated or act out from time to time. The wise staff member or family member will calmly try to divert his attention to something else. Often a change of subject or a change of scenery presented in a friendly non-threatening manner is all that is needed to change disturbing behavior.

Sharing the Care

Forcing someone to do something they don't want to do can be dangerous. My loved one is resistant to doing some things. I tell the staff what those things are and the ways that have been successful for me in dealing with his resistance.

Consider this: Individuals with Alzheimer's disease or a related disorder may be fearful of water, especially showers. If they are frightened and resist, accidents can occur. You may wish to be present the first few times the aides bathe your relative. Your presence can be reassuring to your relative and the persons who are now responsible for bathing him will appreciate your insight into what has worked at home.

Sharing the Care

Body language can be every bit as important as verbal language. My loved one does not converse with me as much as she used to. I'm learning to interpret her facial expressions and body posture.

Consider this: If your relative can no longer hear you, or progressive dementia has affected her ability to speak and respond to speech, you will both learn new methods of communicating needs and thoughts to one another. Just as you are responding to your relative's body language, she is responding to yours. Continue to be reassuring in your movements, gestures, and facial expressions. Show patience and consideration in your mannerisms and you'll both benefit.

Sharing the Care

Textures and surfaces are fascinating—especially in an environment with limited variation. I look for opportunities to bring my loved one a variety of things to handle and look at. When I am choosing decorating fabric or paint colors for my home, I bring the samples in and ask for her opinion.

Consider this: Many fabrics, colors, and textures may be repeated throughout the care facility for efficiency and economy. Unfortunately, this may not be very stimulating for the residents. Old wallpaper books are excellent for activities involving the sensory stimulus of touch. Call your local wall covering stores and ask for any used books they would normally discard. The different designs, colors, and textures are also useful in many craft activities.

Sharing the Care

I'm letting go of the way things used to be. Things change. I need to grow and change too. I accept the present situation. I find joy in new ways. I'm good to myself and to others.

Consider this: The reality of the present may be easier for you to accept and understand than it is for your relative. If your relative is confused, relate to him where he is. Trying to make him understand or stay in the present is not necessary and will be futile and exhausting for both of you. Your reality and his may no longer be the same. Just enjoy the fact that he is content to be in his own space and time.

Sharing the Care

Elderly people often fear being deserted by their family members. My loved one has never expressed this fear, but I make sure he knows I care about him. I am not preoccupied with taking care of him, but I do spend quality time with him. I also remember I have a life, too. Balance is important in both our lives.

Consider this: Your relative needs a healthy balance of friends and family—just like you do. If you monopolize his time, he won't have the opportunity to make friends among his peers in the care facility. You both need a life apart from each other. So, don't feel you have to be with him all the time!

Sharing the Care

It's nice to have something to look forward to when you get up in the morning. Some people just seem to find joy in small things and in things others might overlook. The rest of us might need to look more closely for things that can bring us joy. They're there!

Consider this: Happiness is an attitude. It's a conscious decision we can only make for ourselves. There are plenty of things to look forward to wherever we live or whatever our circumstances. You can help your relative, by being kind and considerate of her, but her happiness is up to her. Don't take responsibility for anyone's happiness—except your own.

Sharing the Care

I try to stay as knowledgeable as possible regarding my loved one's condition. I read the latest medical findings. I attend appropriate support group meetings when I can. I know about the available medical insurance coverage.

Consider this: Even though you may have a doctor who makes calls to the care facility, don't hesitate to ask for a second opinion on important medical procedures. Your relative has the same rights as always. Hopefully he has made his feelings known on life support issues and has provided a health care directive and named someone as health care proxy should he become unable to speak for himself.

Sharing the Care

I'm thankful for a care facility that focuses on the needs of people of all ages. The things they do and the practices they embrace show their concern for everyone's well being.

Consider this: Some progressive facilities provide day care for their employees' children. Not only is this a great service and incentive for the work force, it also provides daily opportunities for inter-generational activities for both the young and the elderly!

Sharing the Care

Sometimes the obvious is easily overlooked. When an organized activity is not in progress, there is a tendency to think nothing is going on. There are a number of things in the facility which keep my loved one's interest. I realize there are also times when she just wants to be quiet and do nothing. I have those times too!

Consider this: Mid-afternoon can be a slow time. People are often sleepy and low on energy. A snack cart can help break monotony. When special activities are not planned, viewing on-going videos offered in the lounge is a pleasant pastime. Cheerful background music provided throughout the building can help perk everyone up.

Sharing the Care

I avoid asking my loved how he is or how things are going because lately his response is negative. I have done everything I can. I have had his medical concerns checked out and I have investigated all his complaints. His negative responses make me feel guilty, but I remember I am not responsible for his attitude. I visit as often as possible and still maintain a life of my own.

Consider this: Ask if pets can be brought into the facility. The administration might want to see up-to-date immunization records and be assured the pet is clean and friendly. Bringing a family pet when you visit might help your relative concentrate on something other than himself and his complaints. It could also help break some monotony and make your time there more pleasant.

Sharing the Care

I'm constantly learning new ways of doing things. New ideas present themselves every day. All I have to do is look around and unique solutions to unique problems appear.

Consider this: Buying appropriate gifts for your relative may be a new challenge now that her living arrangement has changed. Most department stores have ladies' pajamas and lingerie that don't look like sleepwear. The fabric is comfortable and cannot be seen through. The styles are appropriate for residents to wear in the daytime. Some pajamas look just like casual pantsuits. The waists are elastic and the tops usually button up the front. Like sweat suits, they are easy to get in and out of, however they are more stylish than sweat suits.

Sharing the Care

Repetition is not always a bad thing. In fact, it is often necessary. I find myself having to repeat some of the things I say to my loved one. I fight the temptation to become impatient with him.

Consider this: Make sure you are talking clearly enough for your relative. Look at him and have his full attention when you speak. If he is hard of hearing or if he has dementia, you need to speak slowly and directly. If you are giving directions, give only one part at a time. Wait until he does that part. Repeat it if necessary. Then go on to the next part. Your patience and clarity will make a big difference for both of you.

Sharing the Care

Time seems to go by quickly for me, but not always for my loved one. I try to remain sensitive to her need to spend time with me, as well as being true to myself and my other commitments.

Consider this: Most facilities provide every resident with a large monthly activity calendar. Post it in your relative's room and go over the activities with her. Mark the activities she wants to attend. Use a colorful marker. If you have special things you plan to do together, mark those dates also. Some families have had stickers made with individual family member's pictures on them. They stick them on the date they plan to visit next. Seeing the stickers on the calendar gives their relative something to look forward to. A glance at the calendar tells family members what might be a good day for their next visit.

Sharing the Care

My loved one is close to a number of the people he lives with. They converse, share meals, and join together in activities on a daily basis. They give each other emotional support. The affection and concern they have for one another is a beautiful thing to see.

Consider this: Residents often become extended family to one another. They form bonds as strong as college students do in dormitories. If a fellow resident dies, the loss is often felt as profoundly as for family members. Many facilities are aware of this. They hold special memorial services in their own chapel for staff and residents to attend.

Sharing the Care

The care facility is filled with special problems and special needs. The staff comes up with special solutions. It's a big house with a lot of people living in it!

Consider this: Wandering by residents with dementia can present a number of problems. The safety of the wanderer is an obvious one. Protecting the privacy of his neighbors is another. Besides the evident need for security doors to the outside, some facilities have success in using Dutch doors on wanders' rooms. Scheduled supervised walks also help. When rocking chairs are provided, some wanders are content to rock rather than wander. Being registered in a national program and wearing one of their wanderer I.D. bracelets is still appropriate for any resident of a care facility who wanders.

Sharing the Care

I try to do things with my loved one, not for my loved one. I only do the things for him he cannot do for himself. If I do something for him he is perfectly capable of doing himself, I am taking something precious away from him.

Consider this: A person's pride and dignity are precious indeed. Elderly people suffer enough losses without losing the privilege of doing for themselves the things they can still do alone. Independence is very difficult to let go of, whether it is a gradual or sudden loss. We must be sensitive to the losses the elderly experience and let them embrace every bit of remaining independence they have.

Sharing the Care

I don't blame aging for all my loved one's problems. Old age is not a catch-all. He seems to have enough limitations imposed on him in the name of being old. Much of his present behavior has always been part of his personality. Many of the things he experiences are the result of actions he chooses to take. Old age has not made him a different person and it has not made him a victim of some awful curse.

Consider this: If your relative can't hear well, don't assume it's part of old age. Ask his doctor to check for imbedded ear wax. Isn't that the first thing you'd have checked for yourself or a child?

Sharing the Care

A lifetime of habits and preferences need not be changed just because your address has changed. My loved one is used to doing certain things every day—often in a certain way. Some things have had to change because of congregate living, but many do not have to change.

Consider this: When a facility is people-oriented rather than task-oriented, the tasks often get done more efficiently and with less stress on everyone. Some staffs have realized the value in allowing residents to get up each morning when they want to. The residents are given choices of the kinds of breakfasts they prefer and the times. It's much more like living at home and getting up at your own pace. The aides and nurses actually find they get their morning work done on time and the tone for the entire day is more cheerful!

Sharing the Care

Sometimes my loved one tells me she is just a nuisance. I tell her she isn't, but she seems to say it a lot. Is she looking to me for more reassurance of her value to us? Is she searching for more attention and validation?

Consider this: Older people often feel the care they require and receive is an imposition to those who provide it. They may be used to caring and doing for others and are not comfortable being on the receiving end. Make sure the care they receive is given with love. Continue to encourage them to do the things for themselves and others they are still able to do.

Sharing the Care

My loved one gets impatient when his needs aren't met right away. Sometimes he has to wait for someone to answer his calls for assistance.

Consider this: Not having enough staff and the amount of paperwork required by staff members to meet regulations take valuable time away from the hands-on care required by the residents. Both situations can put the staff under pressure. They have the feeling of being rushed all the time. For the most part, administration and staff members try to put the residents and their needs first.

Sharing the Care

One day my loved one told me she felt like she was in prison and had no rights anymore. I had no idea she felt that way. We talked and discussed ways she could retain a sense of control, personal identity, and freedom.

Consider this: Your relative should have the same rights as always—as well as her rights as a resident. In fact, the legal rights of residents should be posted in the care facility. When elderly people need help being moved, dressed, or fed, they are apt to feel they are no longer in control of any aspect of their lives. Participation in the care facility practices and decisions through being a member of the residents' council is a good idea for all residents. It is a way to exercise their rights and retain the control they fear they may have lost.

Sharing the Care

Some residents yell obscenities or call out in a disruptive manner. The staff is good about discouraging it in a positive way by either moving the resident to a quieter area or diverting the resident's interest.

Consider this: Some cognitively impaired residents may become vocally disruptive if they are frightened, in pain, or restricted from doing something they want to do. They may simply misinterpret something someone is doing for them. They should never be punished or ostracized. If they are removed from the room because they are bothering others, it should be done in a cheerful manner by suggesting and introducing a new activity.

Sharing the Care

Change is inevitable. Growth is optional. It isn't change that brings pain and discomfort; it's our resistance to it.

Consider this: If a facility is to continually improve, it must continually change. The administration must keep up with the needs and the latest advancements in an effort to foster the best quality of care possible. Rigidity and inflexibility can be detrimental to all concerned. Acceptance of new ideas, imagination, and a willingness to be open to new possibilities can open all sorts of exciting doors!

Sharing the Care

In my busy life I tend to be looking forward and toward the future. Spending time with and conversing with my loved one is beneficial for me. Reminiscing about the past feels good. It's a refreshing break. We laugh as she retells stories of times I had almost forgotten.

Consider this: Older people are a beautiful link to other times. Details of yesteryears are often more vivid to the elderly than the occurrences of the present day. It can be refreshing indeed to share pleasant memories with them. Relax and enjoy discussing old times with your relative.

Sharing the Care

Timing is important to all of us. We may function better at certain times of the day. Some of us are better in the morning, some in the afternoon or evening. An afternoon nap could be an everyday event or a necessity for some people.

Consider this: If your schedule is flexible, try to determine what time of day is best for your relative to have guests. There may be a time of day he functions best. He might have activities he regularly attends. If you can, take these things into consideration when planning your visits with him.

Sharing the Care

The years of my loved one's increasing dependence upon me brought us closer. Her needs somehow slowed me down and forced me to spend the time with her we hadn't shared in the recent past. If she hadn't needed me, I would have been robbed of the special closeness we now cherish.

Consider this: In parent-child relationships many adult children have long forgotten the closeness of early childhood years. Parents, however, somehow always remember that special time. When caring for an aging parent, a close bond often forms—the roles may change, but the bond becomes strong again.

Sharing the Care

I am doing the best I can at this very moment. There are many demands on me and I have a great number of responsibilities. I must remember to be as good to myself as I am to those I care about.

Consider this: Stress can make anyone sick—emotionally, physically, or both. Excessive guilt and depression can do the same thing. Take as good care of yourself as you do your loved ones. If you are having a distressful time handling any aspect of your caregiving situation, seek professional counseling and get your life back on track. Where does it say you have to carry everything alone on your shoulders?

Sharing the Care

My loved one is afraid of falling. I make sure his glasses are clean and his eyes are checked regularly. His shoes are sturdy and the soles are skid-proof, but he worries about falling nevertheless. At least I know he is careful and takes no chances!

Consider this: To make up for increasing frailty and sensory losses, the elderly depend more and more on their environment. Familiar surroundings and consistent placement of furniture and belongings are extremely important. Lighting can make a big difference in their feeling of security. Well-placed handrails make walking safer.

Sharing the Care

My loved one gives me hope. She has survived so many things in her lifetime. I marvel at her—at the ways she has coped. I share with her the things I am going through in my life. I ask her to share her coping skills with me.

Consider this: Emphasize your relative's strengths by asking for her advice. You may be surprised how much her experience and wisdom can help you. You'll be doing both of you a favor. You'll boost her self-esteem and confidence. And, you'll receive valuable assistance your peers may not be able to give you.

Sharing the Care

My loved one enjoys entertaining children. Her home was filled with things that delighted her grandchildren. The youngsters who visit her now also find delight and have great joy being around her. She just has a way with the little ones.

Consider this: If children visit your relative, bring her things she can give them. Bake cookies using her favorite recipes. Keep safe toys in her room for them. If she can read out loud to them, provide some children's books. Help her make their visits special occasions she and the kids both look forward to.

Sharing the Care

Sometimes I feel guilty because my loved one requires care I cannot give him. I know it's not my fault. So why do I put an added burden on myself? Guilt is just something heavy to carry and I don't need it. I'm going to stop carrying it around. Whenever I am tempted to pick it up, I must tell myself I can't change my loved one's situation. But I can improve my emotional well being by refusing to dwell on guilt.

Consider this: There are things we wish we could do for others that we just can't. Some things are out of our hands and our control. What we can do is offer unconditional love and give quality time in the proper balance and perspective with the rest of our lives and our other relationships.

Sharing the Care

Focusing on reality may no longer be appropriate for my loved one. Past events seem to hold more meaning than recent ones. So, I ask her about her childhood, her schooldays, and her parents. She seems to be confused about current happenings, but is delighted by our conversations about yesteryears.

Consider this: Short-term memory decreases as dementia progresses in people with Alzheimer's disease or related disorders. Stressing the day's date and activities may not be significant to them. Instead, meet them where they are and on their level. Don't try to explain, argue, or force a point.

Sharing the Care

Just as I am concerned with my loved one's comfort, I must know and safeguard my own comfort levels as well. My well being is important too.

Consider this: Don't take advantage of yourself or push yourself beyond your limits. Establish and keep daily rituals that you find comfort in. Caring for someone as you do, can be extremely stressful. Be kind to yourself. Make sure each day contains some activities you enjoy!

Sharing the Care

Loneliness seems to stem from an absence of love and companionship—real or perceived. The loss of lifetime sources of love and companionship can be devastating. I try to give my relative love and companionship. I encourage her to make new friends among other residents who may also be feeling lonely.

Consider this: It takes time to replace and build new support systems. If you find your relative making comparisons between old friends and new ones, remind her that no two situations or times are the same. Suggest ways she could be helping others. People who appear aloof may actually be shy and insecure. Kind encouragement to them from your relative can be the seeds that grow into meaningful new friendships.

Sharing the Care

I rented a wheelchair. I spent the day in it so I could experience what my loved one deals with every day. I was frustrated. I became impatient with myself and with others. I learned a lot. The term *wheelchair-accessible* has new meaning to me now.

Consider this: Even within care facilities numerous changes and adjustments are needed to help those who rely on wheelchairs. One facility was proud of its gardens and encouraged residents to plant seedlings for both indoor and outdoor flower and vegetable beds. They provided wheelchair-accessible planting tables and gardens.

Sharing the Care

A sense of belonging is essential to a person's self-worth and identity. Staff and family members do everything possible to promote this important element in the quality of life for all residents.

Consider this: Many care facilities find value in naming hallways with street names. Living at 101 Orchard Lane is more comforting and inviting than Room 101 in Hallway B. In these hallway areas some facilities have even constructed small indoor front porches at the entry to every resident's room. Flowering plants and rocking chairs are a part of each porch. Residents enjoy sitting on their own porches and visiting neighbors' front porches. Personalized mailboxes on individual porch entrances are also nice additions.

Sharing the Care

I sense a sadness in my loved one lately. A decrease in her stamina is evident also. She is easily overwhelmed by everyday circumstances and occurrences. She doesn't seem to be coping with things like she usually does.

Consider this: Depression can be caused by a number of happenings. A recent illness or operation may bring it on. Loss of appetite, exaggerated worries, trouble sleeping, and preoccupation with physical complaints may all indicate depression. Depression can also cause dementia symptoms. Don't ignore any changes in your relative. Accurate diagnosis and appropriate care are in order at all times.

Sharing the Care

I encourage my loved one to stretch his mind as well as his body. Growing and learning are a part of life. And, my loved one is still living!

Consider this: Many forward-thinking communities offer some of their adult education and extension courses to residents of local care facilities. They hold the classes in the care facility during daytime hours. The interest and response is usually positive. Residents feel good about continuing their education. It's a great opportunity to increase self-esteem.

Sharing the Care

When we lack enthusiasm or hope, our thoughts tend to visit more pleasant times in our past. We retreat from the present. Everyone needs something to look forward to today!

Consider this: Monotony and boredom may manifest themselves in constant weariness and chronic fatigue. The care facility should be providing numerous and varied interests for their residents. Some activities may be planned, but the best ones seem to be implemented as parts of the daily surroundings. The environment should be a pleasant place to wake up to every morning. The atmosphere should be filled with the spontaneous happenings of a busy, cheerful house.

Sharing the Care

I keep a journal. As I re-read some of the entries, my true feelings and concerns become quite evident. I believe it is emotionally healthy for me to continue confiding in my silent, trusted friend.

Consider this: Caring for another person can create stress, which needs to be addressed and dealt with effectively. Frequent entries in a personal journal can be very therapeutic. Also certain patterns may be revealed—both negative and positive ones. Reading our own journals can remind us what has worked in our caregiving journey and what has not. The way we have met challenges along the way can help us with future challenges. We can learn a lot from our journals.

Sharing the Care

My loved one likes to get out of his room as much as possible. The facility offers a number of options available throughout the day. I make sure he knows about all the different activities he can partake of and their locations within the facility.

Consider this: One care facility provides a workshop for its residents. Men and women alike spend time there. Many crafts are created and quality companionship abounds. Continuous supervision is provided when residents with Alzheimer's disease use the workshop. Some repetitious activities such as sanding with a simple piece of sandpaper often provide hours of contentment for someone with dementia.

Sharing the Care

I'm not always sure my relative understands what I'm saying when I talk to her. It's been a long time since she actually conversed with anyone. We don't really know how much she comprehends.

Consider this: If your loved one no longer speaks and doesn't react to what is said to her, don't assume she doesn't understand anything. For your sake and hers, it's a good idea to continue to talk to her like you always have. Share the things that are going on in your life, give her time to speak without embarrassing her, and continue to tell her she is loved. Your naturalness and familiarity will be reassuring to both of you.

Sharing the Care

The care facility administration, residents, and staff do everything they can to establish and maintain a feeling of true community in the building.

Consider this: One caring facility has named the lobby area and front hall "Main Street." Rooms that were previously offices have been remodeled to look like friendly hometown shops. There is a post office for receiving and sending mail. The residents' gift shop, barbershop, beauty shop, snack shop, and sweet shop can all be found on Main Street. A wheelchair-accessible public telephone booth provides another feature for residents and their family members.

Sharing the Care

I'm fairly well organized and I like efficiency. For the most part, I think the care facility runs smoothly. Not much falls through the cracks. My loved one is in pretty good hands!

Consider this: When residents are on an outing with relatives or friends, the facility must be informed—preferably ahead of time. Many facilities post a sign-out book on each unit or at the front desk. When residents are out of the building, the persons responsible for them need to sign them in and out. Many a search party has been formed when family members neglect to do this. Needless to say, the family doesn't build up popularity points with the staff and it's not what team players do!

Sharing the Care

Privacy in congregate living can be an extremely sensitive issue. I respect my loved one's right to his privacy no matter where he lives. Sometimes he has to be firm in his quest for it.

Consider this: Family, staff, and fellow residents need to be especially aware of the need for privacy among all residents. Many facilities have installed doorbells on every room. Sometimes special measures have to be taken to discourage confused residents from overstepping boundaries. Doors can be painted to look like bookshelves. Ribbons can be run across open doorways. Stop signs are often effective. Remember, residents always retain the right to refuse or turn away unwanted visitors.

Sharing the Care

I like things that are user-friendly. Being difficult doesn't make something more sophisticated or more desirable. A business that is run in an easy friendly atmosphere is welcoming.

Consider this: Many facilities have a directory in the front lobby to help visitors locate residents' rooms. Often a pleasant map showing the layout of the physical building and grounds accompanies the directory. The map also helps new guests become acquainted with everything the facility offers. It may even suggest alternative areas to visit in, rather than the residents' rooms.

Sharing the Care

People function better when they are kept informed. Changes in facility personnel, policies, and procedures need to be communicated in a professional manner. The facility's monthly newsletter does a good job of informing everyone who will be affected by any change—staff, residents, and family members.

Consider this: Sometimes staff members change roles and the residents and families need to be aware of the change. The care facility may experience cuts in personnel. When everyone is aware of the cut, alternative ways to get the job done may surface. One home had to reduce the grounds services to the basics of mowing. When the local garden club heard about the cut back, they offered to weed the grounds and care for the plantings as volunteers.

Sharing the Care

The environment my loved one occupies must be as home-like as attainable in this setting. After all, this is her domicile. I will do all I can to help make her surroundings as much like her former homes as possible.

Consider this: Medical equipment, hoyer lifts, and utility carts have no business occupying space in the resident lounges. Staff should avoid using living areas for extra storage room. If you observe this practice, politely inform them of the need for proper storage of these items. The comfort and safety of residents and visitors can also be a factor in discouraging this thoughtless practice.

Sharing the Care

The biggest problem I have with the care facility is what I perceive as inattention to detail. I realize they don't have the number of staff or the time to always give my loved one the individual attention I want him to have. But, I still wish they could be more attentive to the things that are most important to him.

Consider this: Caring personnel are usually sensitive to the details that matter most to residents and their family members. Be sure to let them know if you feel some aspect of care is being neglected. Realize that family and friends provide a great deal of the emotional care and quality time spent with the residents, while the professional caregivers primarily attend to physical needs.

Sharing the Care

The channels of communication in the facility seem to be pretty good. When I have a special request or when some aspect of my loved one's care is altered, word gets around fairly quickly.

Consider this: Communication between staff members is essential. Talking together and sharing important information about residents is always a good idea. Something added to a care plan may not be seen right away, especially by part-time employees. In addition to the written words in the care plan, some employees share new information by posting a note in the resident's room and one in the staff lounge.

Sharing the Care

My loved one has always been on the cutting edge of technology. The physical problems he now experiences don't keep him from exploring and utilizing the modern conveniences and inventions of today.

Consider this: Many care facility residents enjoy having personal laptop computers. They provide hours of enjoyment and interest. The possibilities are limitless. Games can be played, letters written, and new knowledge can be gained. One gentleman created a newsletter for the residents in his facility. Other residents began offering ideas and submitting articles. The newsletter circulated among the residents, staff, and family members. Everyone looked forward to reading it—as well as contributing to it.

Sharing the Care

My loved one counts on me. I want to be reliable. I would not intentionally make him anxious or give him cause for concern. I respect him and I'm careful to follow through on the things I tell him I'll do. I never agree to something—just to humor him.

Consider this: If you tell your relative you will visit at a certain time, make every effort you can to be there and to be on time. If the staff is aware of a planned visit, they usually talk to the resident about it. They often help him get ready to assure him he looks especially nice. Your relative may voluntarily give up a facility activity in anticipation of a visit from you. Make sure you let the facility know if you have to break a date with him. His time is valuable too!

Sharing the Care

I try to acquaint myself with all that goes on in the facility. They offer many varied activities for the residents. I realize most residents look forward to the activities and to certain times of the day. I'm amazed at the variety of activities residents can enjoy every day.

Consider this: When you're cleaning your house and have the urge to throw things out, think of the care facility and some of their needs. The activity director can make use of a number of things. Don't get rid of old games and puzzles without offering them to the facility first. Magazines are great for making collages. Craft items are always in demand.

Sharing the Care

My loved one is proud of me. This doesn't embarrass me. Actually, it's a nice feeling to be loved unconditionally. He enjoys introducing me to his friends. He even brags about me occasionally and I realize he's earned the right.

Consider this: Try to attend the special functions the facility plans. Your relative will be happy to have you there. Notice the residents who have no family in attendance and encourage them to sit with your family. Bring your camera along and offer to take pictures of the event—the decorations, the food, and the people! When they are developed, make your photos available to all who participated.

Sharing the Care

None of us are at our best when we're tired. Tempers get short and we become irritable. Patience tends to disappear.

Consider this: Evenings can be an especially hectic time in a care facility. Many residents need two people assisting them to get ready for bed. Residents become cranky waiting for their turn. Overcoming this difficult time of day is a challenge for staff and residents. Soft music piped through the facility, volunteers serving decaffeinated after-dinner coffees, and videos of old comedy movies playing in the lounge, can all help make it a more pleasant time for everyone.

Sharing the Care

My loved one is confused and he doesn't always know who I am. But I keep on visiting him. It makes me feel better and I hope my visits are good for him too.

Consider this: People suffering from Alzheimer's disease or a related disorder don't always recognize their family members. They shouldn't be put on the spot or asked if they know who someone is. In fact, it helps to identify you and others in a normal non-threatening manner by saying something like, "Hi Dad! Here we are—your adoring daughters, Carol and Betty. Hope you're as glad to see us today as we are to see you." This should help put everyone at ease.

Sharing the Care

Each one of us is a special gift to the world. When gifts go unnoticed, we miss something meant to be cherished and enjoyed. I realize my loved one's unique qualities. He may have some problems right now, but what a gift he is to us!

Consider this: Treating someone with appreciation and realizing how wonderfully unique they are can make a big difference in the way they see themselves. It may even influence the way they ultimately view life. Every resident of the care facility needs someone to say hello to them, to spend quality time with them, to get to know them, and to appreciate them.

Sharing the Care

Devotional readings, meditating on scriptures, and prayer time are an important part of my loved one's life. Due to physical handicaps he is no longer able to do some of these things by himself. Now we do them together.

Consider this: Reading to your relative is a wonderful activity. And, don't forget many inspirational books are available on audio tapes. When you are not there, ask the staff to play them for your relative. This is an important part in the life of someone who is accustomed to daily readings and devotionals.

Sharing the Care

I take my caregiving responsibilities seriously. My loved one may be living in a care facility now, but I am still very involved with her and the care she receives. I don't want to be left in the dark about anything concerning her well being.

Consider this: Many family members complain they aren't told when their relative's physician makes visits and they never get an update on their relative's health. If this is true for you, let the doctor know your needs. If your phone calls to him are not returned, send your request by mail. If you receive no response, consider changing physicians.

Sharing the Care

When I was a child I hated being told I had to eat something I didn't like. Or, being forced to finish everything on my plate when I was full and didn't want to eat any more. As an adult, I can't imagine someone making me do these things.

Consider this: Many long-term care facilities realize their residents have less and less control over some aspects of their lives. So, in an attempt to preserve adult dignity, they try to give the residents as many choices as possible. Within the realm of safety, they avoid making unnecessary restrictions and rules. They acknowledge and respect the fact this is a home inhabited by adults.

Sharing the Care

My loved one is reserved and tends to be reclusive. She has never been social. Being surrounded by other people now is difficult for her.

Consider this: Some residents resent what they view as a constant barrage of intruders. They feel everyone knows their business and everyone gets into their things. Protecting privacy and personal space is a hard thing to do in a congregate living situation. Look for ways to help your relative achieve a more comfortable degree of privacy within the facility and within her reasonable need for care.

Sharing the Care

Due to circumstances and distance, I am unable to be with my loved one as often as I would like. This prohibits me from doing many of the daily or weekly things I would normally do for him.

Consider this: Some facilities have assembled a group of volunteers from churches or other organizations who perform a shopping service for residents who cannot go out and don't have relatives nearby. Individual volunteers are assigned to individual residents. The volunteers go through local newspaper ads with the residents and shop for any items they may want or need for themselves. They also help them select and purchase gifts for their family and friends. Close trusting friendships usually evolve.

Sharing the Care

The residents in our facility have achieved a strong feeling of community. They've become a team. They take pride in the name of their home. They work together to achieve goals.

Consider this: A community with a number of care facilities has instituted an annual Golden Olympics. Residents of the participating facilities work, plan, and practice for the event all year long. Matching T-shirts for team members are purchased, banners are made, and picnic food is planned. Events include spelling bees, baking contests, wheelchair races, relays, beanbag tosses, and shuffle board. Participants receive ribbons. The facility that wins the most categories proudly houses and displays the coveted winner's trophy until the next year.

Sharing the Care

I cannot be all things to all people. I am just one person. At times I feel my family responsibilities put too many demands on me. I want to be fair to everyone—including myself.

Consider this: If you are constantly giving out and not getting any self-fulfillment or any rest, you will become empty and exhausted. You won't be able to help anyone, not even yourself. Be realistic about the things you can and cannot do and the amount of things you try to do. You need to take as good care of yourself as you do everyone else—or you'll not have anything in you to give others.

Sharing the Care

I love my elderly relative, but I must admit sometimes I resent the extra time and effort his care involves. I don't really have much free time and a great deal of what I do have revolves around him and his care.

Consider this: Stand back and look at your situation objectively and realistically. Perhaps you're doing more than your relative requires or expects. You may be overdoing because deep down you expect it of yourself, or you feel guilty if you don't do a lot. Maybe you are the one putting unrealistic demands on yourself. You might need a small vacation away. Take a break and be good to yourself!

Sharing the Care

There is a refreshing new child-like quality in my loved one. She is delighted by everything. Small pleasures abound everywhere.

Consider this: It's fun, easy, and inexpensive to bring little gifts when you visit. Favorite sweets, costume jewelry, a cheery coffee mug, or a single flower usually bring joy to their recipients. Unexpected gifts and the exultation they institute have no age limits. They may provide the lift your relative and your visits need. Your thoughtfulness will surely make your relative feel special and convey your love for her.

Sharing the Care

Small changes in the environment are good for all of us. Variety in some things can truly be the spice of life. Routine and familiarity are fine, but we all need some cheerful changes once in a while or the space we inhabit can become awfully dull.

Consider this: When doing seasonal or holiday decorating for your relative's room, don't forget the bed afghan, throw, or lap robe. Today they all come in washable fabrics. Numerous prints, colors, and seasonal themes abound. Specialty throw pillows are always a delight. They're available in many shapes—pumpkins and apples, hearts and roses. Change them often! The gaiety they provide is sure to perk up the room and the resident.

Sharing the Care

No one likes to be ignored. Lately my loved one seems to be ignoring some of the things I say to her. I'm trying to figure out if she is hard of hearing or is exercising selective hearing.

Consider this: If the physician has ruled out hearing problems, make sure you are giving your relative plenty of time to respond to what you say. Consider the content of your conversations. Perhaps you are talking about things she doesn't want to talk about or has no interest in. Conversely, some residents feel what they say is ignored by staff and family. If your relative has expressed this concern, speak to the staff about it. If your relative is able to attend the resident council meetings, suggest she do so.

Sharing the Care

Communication is an essential element for human beings. Without it we feel lost and isolated. When we cannot rely on verbal communications, we must become creative in finding and utilizing other sources. I've observed many innovative forms of communication throughout the facility.

Consider this: A large magnetic alphabet board is a great addition to anyone's room. Its uses and benefits are many. Staff and family can post reminders of daily events on it. A resident who is unable to speak can use it as a means of communication. Often Alzheimer's patients enjoy spelling their names and using it for information they have retained.

Sharing the Care

Before I attend my loved one's health care meetings, I make notes of the things I want to discuss. I often have concerns or suggestions. Sometimes other members of the family have questions, cares, or ideas they want me to bring up. Right after the meeting I usually write them a brief account of what was discussed and what I believe was accomplished.

Consider this: Make sure the care facility has a copy of your relative's Medicare and supplemental health insurance cards on file. They should also have copies of all health care directives and should be informed of any special and specific family requests such as wanting an autopsy upon the death of your loved one.

Sharing the Care

My loved one's world is smaller and less complicated than it once was. When I visit him I rather enjoy entering his world and leaving my complicated one behind. We talk of simple things. For me it's a bittersweet joy.

Consider this: Progressive dementia of the Alzheimer's type usually takes its captives back to simpler times and things. If we learn to communicate with them on their level and try to glimpse the world as they see it and join them for brief moments, who knows what comfort and peace we may be giving them— and perhaps ourselves as well.

Sharing the Care

We're fortunate to have a number of family members living near the care facility. This helps take the burden off any one person and it makes visits easier and more fun.

Consider this: Some large families try to schedule monthly suppers together in the care facility's private family dining room. They all bring in favorite family dishes. Their loved one enjoys a variety of foods she doesn't usually get in the main dining room. When large families come together, the range in ages and the liveliness of activity generally create a good time for everyone who attends.

Sharing the Care

Eating has become more and more difficult for my loved one. Sometimes he chokes. Sometimes he even refuses to eat. I know we are all doing everything we can. The staff and I both try to help feed him and encourage him, but it takes forever—and most of the food remains on the plate.

Consider this: Feeding is an especially difficult issue for persons in the advanced stages of Alzheimer's disease. Food with a special consistency might be required and lots of staff time is often necessary to individually feed them. Cues may have to be given to encourage chewing and swallowing. Keeping the resident's attention on eating can be a challenge. Liquefied food supplements offered frequently during the day might help insure proper nutrition.

Sharing the Care

My loved one's behavior can be a problem if he is frightened, frustrated, or scolded. The attitude of those around him and the physical environment he inhabits have a great influence on his behavior. If people are accepting of him and his environment is easy and pleasing to him, he generally reacts accordingly.

Consider this: When someone's needs are not met, problematic behavior can occur. In care facilities, staff must learn to meet the needs of residents cheerfully and creatively. Patient rights must be observed and maintained at all times.

Sharing the Care

I am constantly looking for new and creative ways to make a difficult situation easier. The whole family, including our elderly loved one, has accepted the reality of the need for the care facility. Now we concentrate on making the best of each day and each visit.

Consider this: Taking one day at a time and enjoying it to the fullest is excellent advice for every life situation. The care facility is no exception. If residents, staff, and family members all remembered to do this every day, the environment would be one filled with smiling faces. Smiles are contagious. Try spreading yours around!

Sharing the Care

I'm familiar with the term *peace of mind*. But, lately my loved one has been talking about how she feels in her heart. I'm beginning to think that *peace of heart* is a reality.

Consider this: You may find there are things your elderly relative just has to talk about. She may say things like, "I want to tell you what's on my heart." They will usually be things that go deeper than things that are just on her mind. Whatever she chooses to call them, they are subjects of great significance and concern to her. Listen to her. Don't put her off. She needs to talk to you about them while she can. She trusts you with something that is obviously important to her.

Sharing the Care

Breaks from reality and routine are good for all of us. I need to break out once in a while and get silly. Dressing up in a costume may be just what I need. Maybe the people around me need it, too!

Consider this: Parties and costumes can make even the grumpiest residents grin. Most facilities decorate for Halloween, but colorful autumn decorations of pumpkins and leaves are always more appreciated than scary or spooky decorations. Staff and family members dressed in non-threatening costumes passing out safe edible goodies can help create a fun time for everyone. Visits from school children in costumes always delight residents.

Sharing the Care

Some days I just don't have time to get everything done. I find I must make good use of every waking moment. I want to visit my loved one, but it takes time I don't always have.

Consider this: If you have a portable task to do that can be done while you sit, consider doing it when you visit with your relative. As long as you won't be ignoring him and can still carry on a conversation while you work on your project, it may help the time go faster for you. It could also provide a new subject to talk about. It might interest him and he may even offer to help you!

Sharing the Care

My loved one's physical strength and endurance is naturally not what it used to be. Nevertheless, I am concerned about what I perceive as continued lack of stimulation and use. When I am with him, I encourage him to move and exercise his body as much as he can.

Consider this: Physical inactivity takes its toll on the body. Even mild exercising can greatly benefit and increase muscle strength. Make sure your relative is getting some beneficial daily exercise. If you are concerned, talk to the physical therapist and the activity director to determine what is appropriate for your relative.

Sharing the Care

A sense of loss pervades my loved one. Without speaking it, the word *loss* seems to permeate her existence. I don't want it to overwhelm her. I am constantly looking for ways to help her compensate or overcome the heavy sense of loss she is experiencing.

Consider this: Remaining strengths can come through creative arts. Art therapy might do wonders to overcome your relative's losses. She may feel she's lost control over many aspects of her life. Through the freedom of art she will have control over designs, colors, shapes, and subjects. Residents who have lost language skills or communication skills often express themselves through their art.

Sharing the Care

My loved one takes his privileges and responsibilities seriously. He has always been a good citizen. He is proud of his country.

Consider this: If your relative is mentally competent he should naturally be a part of local and national elections. Take him to vote or ask the staff if they have made provisions to transport residents to the nearest polling place. Make sure your relative is registered with his new address. Absentee voting may also be a possibility, but must be done well in advance of the election date.

Sharing the Care

Since I don't live near my loved one, I worry about him and I put myself under a heavy blanket of guilt. I write to him a lot. It helps us keep in touch and makes me feel better. I visit whenever I can get away, but unfortunately that's not very often.

Consider this: Being a long-distance caregiver to someone in a care facility is no easier than being right next-door. In fact, the frustrations and the self-imposed guilt can be worse. Thankfully, today there are many caring professionals and volunteers who can ease a family's anxieties and serve as an extended family for the resident. Be aware of the help that is available and make use of it for your peace of mind and your relative's quality of care.

Sharing the Care

My loved one has always had empathy for what others are going through. She understands difficult times and reaches out when someone is in need. Despite her limitations and handicaps, this beautiful quality still shines as bright as ever.

Consider this: Resident volunteers in one facility have formed a wonderful bond with elderly shut-ins in their town. The participating residents are each matched up with a shut-in. The residents make daily telephone calls to check if they are okay and to chat for a few moments. They each have an emergency number to call if they get no answer or if they believe there is a problem.

Sharing the Care

My loved one looks to family for the support and unconditional love we can supply. We see the appreciation in his eyes when we are able to do little acts of love and kindness for him.

Consider this: Check your relative's fingernails and toenails to see if they are being cared for. You may want to bring a nail file and clippers with you when you visit. Soaking nails in warm water before cutting or clipping always makes the job easier. If you prefer not to do the toenails, the services of a visiting podiatrist should be available. Just let the staff know of the need. Massaging feet and hands with warm lotion is always a caring gesture. Family members may be the only ones who have the time for this thoughtful expression of love.

Sharing the Care

I let my loved one know I enjoy his company. I try not to appear rushed when we visit. I listen. I look into his eyes when we talk. I take his hands in mine.

Consider this: Even if your relative is confused or suffers from a form of dementia, you can have comforting and interesting visits. Looking at pictures of past shared experiences, initiating reminiscent conversation, or bringing in a simple craft project similar to ones you have done together in the past, can be reassuring. But, don't forget—just being there is what's important!

Sharing the Care

No matter how good the facility is, there are things my loved one misses. I try to be aware of what they are and when possible I supply them myself.

Consider this: Cooking meals for large numbers often eliminates the presence of fresh fruit and vegetables. Most are frozen or canned and often overcooked. Family members can bring in fresh items as snacks. Vegetable juice from health food stores is refreshing and nourishing. Make sure there is plenty of liquid and fiber in your relative's diet.

Sharing the Care

I listen to what my loved one has to say. She has much wisdom. I ask her opinion on issues. I consider her advice when I have an important decision to make. I let her know she still has a special importance and place in my life. I learn a lot from her.

Consider this: Many older people consider what they say before they speak. Allow your relative time to respond to questions or comments you make. Give her adequate time to enter into a conversation. Show your interest in hearing from her. There will usually be much thought and wisdom behind what she says, if you show her proper consideration and respect. Rushing or showing impatience will not enhance visits or promote good feelings. Taking time will be time well spent!

Sharing the Care

The ability to be creative does not necessarily diminish with age. I am delightfully amazed at the things residents in our facility come up with. More power to them!

Consider this: Based on past interests, one resident council has formed weekly clubs for residents to attend. Many are planned for late afternoon and early evening when things seem to drag. Bridge, knitting, quilting, chess, and garden clubs are among the most popular. They invite experts to come speak to them. One club meets solely for entertainment and advertises in the local newspaper for amateur comedians, musicians, and playgroups to come entertain them.

Sharing the Care

A second of cheerfulness goes a long way! It takes no longer to say hello in a cheery manner than in a grumpy one. I observe how the staff at all levels greet the residents they pass in the hall. Believe it or not, some don't even acknowledge the residents they pass by!

Consider this: Being constantly ignored is one of the worst things a person can endure. Staff may be super busy and just need a friendly reminder. Try voicing your concern in a non-judgmental way. Perhaps by saying, "My relative loves to be acknowledged. Could you just pop your head in his room when you go by and say hi? Or give him a pat on the arm when you see him in the hall? I know it will mean a lot to him."

Sharing the Care

I can be right or I can be close. Occasionally, I'm even wrong. But I give everything my best try. Sometimes I'm right on the first try—sometimes I'm not even close. Even so, I'm giving life my best and I won't give up!

Consider this: When planning family celebrations in the facility, remember the staff generally begins getting residents ready for bed early in the evening. Your relative is most likely used to going to bed fairly early. She's probably tired in the evenings. If sun downing is an issue, celebrations should definitely be in the daytime. Saturday or Sunday afternoons may work out best for most members of your family.

Sharing the Care

Some old fashioned remedies really work. I've learned many of them from my elderly loved one. She smiles in approval when I suggest doing some of the things she has taught me. Most of it makes sense and is worth passing on!

Consider this: Tired eyes can be temporarily brightened by placing cotton balls soaked in milk on closed eyelids for a few minutes. Mint tea can sweeten breath and help digestion. Consider the use of natural stool softeners for relief of constipation before resorting to harsh laxatives. These may be things your relative is used to and she will recognize as gentle natural ways of caring.

Sharing the Care

Because of dementia my loved one often exhibits repetitive behavior. She rolls and re-rolls the hem of the tablecloth, folds a piece of paper in tiny squares, and taps her leg with her hand over and over again. She sure has a lot of energy. She keeps her focus on the same action for a long time.

Consider this: Try making an activity apron for your relative. Attach objects to a vinyl apron. A plastic spoon and dish, a large plastic zipper, plastic rings intertwined, and big buttons to be buttoned and unbuttoned can be safely attached to the apron. It will provide hours of activity and energy release.

Sharing the Care

My loved one has the right not to be deceived. Our family is as honest with her as we always have been. We include her in all decisions about her care—the big ones and the little ones. Since she is coherent and competent, we won't shield her from truths regarding her health.

Consider this: An elderly person who is mentally capable of discussing her own care and health issues deserves the right to know all the facts and make decisions regarding her care and treatments. When this is done, the family is greatly relieved of guilt issues and closer bonds form. Openness and honesty are healthy for all concerned. She should have a healthcare proxy and healthcare directives already signed should she become unable to make decisions.

Sharing the Care

Caregiving of my elderly loved one just seemed to fall into my lap. Maybe it's because I usually take charge or because I live the closest. Perhaps I had a need to prove my love—or get approval. But now that I'm left with all the responsibility I feel my efforts are taken for granted by everyone.

Consider this: Shared decisions usually work out the best. But, it's never too late. Call a meeting of all your family members. If you live far apart, arrange for a conference call. Be specific with them about ways you need their help. Don't harbor resentments against them because you think they should be doing more. To them it may seem like you have everything under control. They may not know how to contribute without your suggestions and your invitation to help.

Sharing the Care

There are days when my loved one seems listless and not at all like her usual self. I don't push her on those days. I don't give her pep talks. I sit quietly and hold her hand.

Consider this: Become knowledgeable of the interactions of certain drugs. If you are concerned about a combination of medications or that your loved one may be over-medicated or unnecessarily medicated, talk to the head nurse and to her physician. It's always a good idea to periodically check her medications.

Sharing the Care

Through expressing gentleness and caring I've actually become stronger emotionally. I'm able to do things I couldn't do before I undertook this caregiving role. In an odd way, I've also found peace with and within myself.

Consider this: When we're helping others and giving of ourselves we often find ourselves. A peace we have been seeking comes to us when we least expect it. Perhaps we've been looking for it in all the wrong places until now. Touching others selflessly with compassionate acts of love promotes personal growth and brings with it an inner peace.

Sharing the Care

The holiday time of the year is fast approaching. I am filled with a number of mixed emotions. A lot of things have changed. It's obvious some traditions will have to be altered. But, with love and consideration of everyone involved, our family may experience a very meaningful holiday season.

Consider this: If you plan on taking your relative to a family member's home for a holiday meal or celebration, plan ahead. Let the staff know days before the event. If you need it, arrange for special transportation well in advance. Remember to get instructions from the staff, should daily medications need to be administered while your relative is out of the facility.

Sharing the Care

Just because we have to readjust some traditions, doesn't mean we can't have a good time. New traditions can be just as meaningful as old ones. I'm thankful for a family that is willing to be flexible when circumstances merit changes.

Consider this: If you are going to be joining your relative for a holiday meal in the facility dining room, let the staff know in plenty of time. Some families arrange for the use of a special family dining room or lounge area for their celebrations. Meals can be catered or the food brought in by family members. Family get-togethers in the facility work well when the resident cannot or does not care to leave the facility.

Sharing the Care

Finding a quiet place to visit within the facility is not always easy. I look forward to peaceful time alone with my loved one. I know he does, too. When the weather is not conducive to going outdoors, we often sit and watch the birds outside his window.

Consider this: Some facilities have noisy and intrusive intercom or loudspeaker systems. They often distract and confuse residents. They interrupt conversations, naps, and visits. Switching to individual pagers for all staff members might prove to be a less offensive alternative. Restaurants successfully use beepers for their servers. Why couldn't all members of the staff use them in care facilities?

Sharing the Care

Flexibility has come to mean a great deal to me. I don't expect perfection and I don't have unrealistic expectations of myself or anyone else. It's really quite freeing!

Consider this: When you plan something special for a visit, be prepared to change in mid-stream. Your relative may not always respond in the way you anticipate. Or, he may respond for a while, lose interest, or change his attention to something else. Be prepared to redirect yours too. It's also not a bad idea to have some alternate plans or activities in mind to suggest to your relative if things get dull.

Sharing the Care

Sometimes I'm overwhelmed by my own emotions. I feel sad about the current circumstances. I know I'm doing everything I can, however it still hurts to see someone suffering or unhappy. I show him a happy face, but often I'm suffering silently too.

Consider this: You need to address your own discomfort as well as your relative's. Your emotional health is of utmost importance. Your inner pain is real, just like your relative's. Be good to yourself. Talk about your feelings with someone you trust and understands the situation, such as the facility chaplain, your own pastor, or another caregiver.

Sharing the Care

I am surprised at the number of families I talk with who are reluctant to voice any concerns or problems they have with the facility administration. They seem to be afraid of compromising the care their family member does get. They fear retaliation against their loved one if they point out policies, practices, omissions, or staff conduct that concerns them.

Consider this: It may be difficult to admit that the care facility is ultimately a business. But, this means your relative is the ultimate customer. A service is being rendered and paid for. The consumer has a right to be satisfied with the product. Your relative may not necessarily move out when dissatisfied, however problems certainly need to be addressed to the administration—and acceptable solutions worked out!

Sharing the Care

One day my loved one stopped recognizing me. He began crying and saying my name and asking where I was. I tried to explain to him that I was right there. Then I realized that didn't help. His dementia had progressed to the point of not recognizing me as me.

Consider this: Attempts to convince him of your identity will only frustrate both of you. You'll both feel better if you say something like, "I'm sorry you're missing her today, but I'm so glad we're together. I do know she loves you very much—just like I do!" Then take his hand and introduce a new activity, preferably something pleasant such as taking a walk with him and stopping for ice cream or candy in the facility's sweet shop.

Sharing the Care

In the world of long-term care facilities little things mean so much. The way people treat each other can make or break someone's day. The manner in which my relative talks to and treats the aides and nurses is as important as the way they are with her. Abusive behavior or abusive speech by anyone is unacceptable.

Consider this: There are not a lot of emotional rewards for residents or staff. Both are surrounded by illness and problems. They may be the problems of old age or over-work. There is not much to rejoice over. When an attitude of mutual respect is shared, common courtesies abound. Consideration of others can make the difference between a dreary place to live and work or a place filled with smiles and small joys. Respect is a two-way street.

Sharing the Care

My loved one always makes the best of any situation she is in. She also cares a great deal for others and seems to understand when someone else may be going through a difficult time.

Consider this: An active resident council is not just for the purpose of voicing complaints. There are many councils that greatly add to the success of the facility. Some have an orientation committee for new residents. Members of the committee help welcome and acquaint new residents with the facility. They chat regularly with the newcomers and answer any questions they may have. They make a point of being friendly. Their caring attention makes a positive difference in the adjustment process for new residents.

Sharing the Care

I try to keep eye contact with my loved one whenever I'm with him. Doing so maintains our communication. I also sit directly across from him, rather than next to him.

Consider this: Looking into someone's eyes certainly shows you care. As a caregiver this can mean also making sure your care recipient's sight is the best it can be. If your relative wears eyeglasses, yearly visits to or from his eye doctor will assure his prescription is up-to-date. Also be aware many people throughout the day handle his glasses. They are on and off for bathing, dressing, and undressing. The frames may have to be adjusted often. Having an extra pair on hand is a good idea.

Sharing the Care

Insincere flattery never really fools anyone—especially mature adults. I want people to talk to my loved one with sincerity and thoughtfulness. It's an important part of the quality care I expect for him.

Consider this: Most elderly people are accustomed to respect and being treated as adults. If you hear aides or nurses calling your relative by inappropriate pet names, nicely tell them what he is used to being called. Care recipients should not be treated like children. Baby talk can be quite insulting to grown adults. And, incontinence undergarments should never be referred to as diapers!

Sharing the Care

I do everything I can to keep my loved one in the holiday swing of things. We continue to do the festive things together she can enjoy. I am sensitive to any limitations she may have.

Consider this: If your relative doesn't shop outside the facility and wants to purchase holiday gifts, consider bringing in catalogs for her to go through. After she's made her selections, you can place the orders for her over the phone. Have them sent to your home. When it's time to wrap them, bring them to her and do it together during one of your visits. She will feel much more a part of the season if she is actively involved.

Sharing the Care

Visits from family and friends are a meaningful part of my loved one's life. They provide many links for him—links to the past, present, and future. They keep him connected to his family and his community. He looks for visitors.

Consider this: Many family members tell friends and clergy to gently awaken their relative if they find him asleep when they call. Likewise, if the resident is not in his room, they should ask a member of the staff where he is and go look for him. Nothing is more disappointing to a care facility resident than to learn he missed a visitor who came when he was sleeping or away from his room!

Sharing the Care

There are a number of holiday preparations my loved one and I still do together. Planning them is as much fun as doing them. I bring in goodies for us to eat while we work. Sometimes we listen to holiday music. It sets the mood.

Consider this: Sending and receiving holiday greeting cards may be something your relative wants to continue. She might need help in the selection of cards, the purchase of stamps, and compiling the list of recipients. If she is unable to write, volunteer to write messages for her. Do all this during your visits. The names of friends and relatives on the list might bring back happy memories and prompt reminiscent conversations.

Sharing the Care

My loved one has Alzheimer's disease and many of the things I take in stride can be upsetting to him. I watch to see how he responds or reacts to changes in his environment. I don't push him to do things he is uncomfortable with or that cause his behavior to change in an adverse manner.

Consider this: The holidays can be a trying time for anyone. Dementia residents may be easily frustrated or overwhelmed by too many festivities. Changing the placement of furniture to accommodate decorations is not a good idea. Be sensitive to the fact parties might be too much for someone who is easily confused. Large crowds, strange foods, and excessive decorations could cause problems.

Sharing the Care

I've made a conscious decision not to get over-involved in commitments outside my normal everyday ones. And, they are quite enough right now. I pick and choose any additional activities carefully. I make sure I have some time for enjoyment and a little free time for myself.

Consider this: As a caregiver, it's imperative you learn to take as good care of yourself as you do your care recipient. Make sure there is time for some relaxation, physical exercise, and fun in your life. This will greatly help you avoid illness, stress, and resentment. Don't over-extend yourself.

Sharing the Care

I probably know my loved one better than anyone else does. As she becomes less able to care for herself I remind myself to be even more attentive to her needs, especially the unspoken ones.

Consider this: No matter how caring the staff is, they don't know your relative like you do. They also have many chores to perform in a specific time frame. Some small individual needs can be inadvertently overlooked. There might be things your loved one can no longer do for herself, but she hasn't told you or the staff. You may want to clean your relative's eyeglasses each time you visit. If you're not sure her dentures are soaked every night, nicely remind the staff of the need.

Sharing the Care

My loved one is more sentimental than he used to be. His eyes tear up easily when he talks. I've learned to listen with my heart as well as my ears. I affirm his life has been meaningful.

Consider this: Tears do not always indicate sorrow. Memories often bring tears of joy and appreciation. Reminiscing seems to be a healthy part of the aging process. Perhaps it's the natural course of being at peace with a lifetime—the good times and the difficult times. Many elders quietly and inwardly reflect on their lives as they prepare for their final days. Journeys of the heart differ from depression. If you are close to your relative, you will most likely recognize the difference.

Sharing the Care

The more my loved one can do for herself and the longer she can do it means a great deal to her. Her self-esteem and her attitude seem to be in direct proportion to her freedom to do things—when and how she wants to!

Consider this: The way a resident's private bathroom is set up can make a big difference in her independence. Grab bars should be near the toilet and the shower or tub. Emergency call buttons must be easily reached from both locations. Raised toilets should be available if needed. Make sure call bells are immediately answered by staff. They should never be turned off at the nurses' station without being investigated in person.

Sharing the Care

When I'm with my loved one, I focus on enjoying our time together. I try not to get bogged down with the realities of the progression of his illness. I am not in denial. I have accepted reality. I do, however make the best of the time we spend with each other.

Consider this: An Alzheimer's patient may move his feet a lot. Turn on lively music so active feet can dance or tap to the music— even from a sitting position. Hands that are constantly in motion may enjoy clapping to music. Spontaneous activities like these often bring joy and smiles. Look for opportunities to incorporate some of the repetitious things he does into enjoyable activities for both of you.

Sharing the Care

When I am inattentive or preoccupied, I miss things I may never get the chance to be a part of again. Each moment is irreplaceable. Every person is irreplaceable. My complete and undivided attention to the people in my life and the moments I share with them are unique gifts to both of us. I'll slow down and savor these precious gifts.

Consider this: Probably the best gift we can give someone who resides in a long-term care facility is our undivided attention when we are with them. Everyone is special and needs to know that they are. The most effective way to reassure someone of this is by our actions. Spending time focusing on your loved one and being genuinely present will be more appreciated than anything else you do for her.

Sharing the Care

Lately my loved one seems to be working her way through a life review. I feel privileged when she shares it with me and I encourage her to do so. It's healthy for both of us. I've learned a great deal about her and about living. It's made me aware that growth never stops.

Consider this: If you sense your relative has an unresolved life event and she seems troubled and unable to resolve it, enlist the help of a trained counselor. Don't waste time, if she hasn't worked through it by now, professional assistance is most likely needed. The facility may provide confidential counseling for residents. Or, a trusted clergy member of your relative's choice may be most appropriate.

Sharing the Care

The holidays elicit varying responses and memories for all of us, depending on our individual observances, traditions, and beliefs. The care facility has residents with diverse backgrounds and cultures. The holidays in this big extended family are educational indeed.

Consider this: Many countries of origin are represented among residents. One family council hosted an unusual holiday party taking the birthplace or background of each resident into account. Wherever possible, they displayed and talked about unique traditions and decorations. Special pastries and ethnic holiday foods were featured. The celebration is now an annual event.

Sharing the Care

Some belongings seem to get lost or misplaced on a fairly regular basis in the care facility. I'm careful not to point fingers. I don't over-react when something is missing— I just help look for it!

Consider this: Some residents mistake items for theirs and walk off with them. Staff may inadvertently place something in the wrong room. People with dementia often hide things. Staff and family members, who know the favorite hiding places, save a great deal of time by looking there first. Family caregivers often purchase inexpensive duplicates of commonly misplaced items.

Sharing the Care

Many of the things I take for granted are no longer possible for or available to my loved one. I try to be sensitive to this reality. Small pleasures have taken on larger meanings. I rejoice in finding ways to help bring these pleasures into her life.

Consider this: Sunshine and fresh air are essential to life. When a frail elder or a terminally ill person is confined to bed, they are often deprived of these important elements. For bedridden individuals, the warmth of sunshine on the skin and the smell of fresh air need not be things of the past. Many facilities have doors, hallways, and ramps wide enough for beds to be rolled to sunny windows or to outdoor garden areas when the weather permits. Don't forget to display pleasing pictures of the outdoors on the walls of your loved one's room.

Sharing the Care

I get overwhelmed by feeling responsible for my elderly loved one. I find relief when I can openly discuss plans with him that directly concern him.

Consider this: If your relative is not confused and does not have dementia, he most likely knows what is best for him and respects his own limitations and fatigue level. If an important family celebration such as a wedding or a graduation is being planned and he is able to leave the facility for outings, ask him to be honest with you. Does he wish to attend? You may find he wants to go to the ceremony, but feels the reception would be too much for him. Honor his decision and make the appropriate and necessary accommodations.

Sharing the Care

It's a privilege to be sharing this gentle time with my loved one. We both sense our time together is growing short. Sometimes we can talk about it—other times we just hold hands and our hearts talk to each other.

Consider this: The ending of a life is a very private matter, yet it can be shared in many meaningful ways with those closest to us. Putting things in order does not necessarily mean financially. Relationships to each other and especially to God are the important issues. If you sense your relative is fearful of death, arrange for a visit with a member of the clergy. Read reassuring scriptures to your relative. Pray with him.

Sharing the Care

It's definitely winter and the seasons have come full cycle. Although the weather is cold, there is comforting warmth indoors. So it is in our hearts. Time has brought a warm glow that radiates within us.

Consider this: Life is easier when we enjoy all the seasons and accept change. Nothing ever remains the same. Change is reality. Resistance to it is futile and brings pain. Those who enjoy life to its fullest know that change is an intricate part of living. Life goes on beyond change and beyond our comprehension of it.

Sharing the Care

I know the value in maintaining a healthy balance between caring for my loved one and meeting my own needs. If I am consumed with his problems and how they affect me, he will become distressed. He may blame himself.

Consider this: Most elderly people fear being a burden to their family more than they fear death. The more relaxed you are with your relative and the more accepting of his current situation, he will be less apt to feel he's a burden to you. He'll know if you're pretending. The secret lies in your ability to remain emotionally healthy and to not become overwhelmed while helping him through this part of his life.

Sharing the Care

Patience certainly has its place in the care facility environment. When people are dependent on others, patience is a critical element. My loved one must patiently wait for my visits. He waits for someone to answer his call button. The aide waits for him to chew his food before offering another spoonful. I walk patiently at his pace when I walk with him.

Consider this: Residents who are impatient have a more difficult time adjusting to the fact staff has many residents to care for. Needs don't always get met immediately. Staff must be patient with the slow pace of the elderly. Patience ought to be practiced by one and all. Understanding of others can stamp out impatience and selfishness.

Sharing the Care

   Laughter and a great sense of humor have always been an integral part of my loved one's personality. She doesn't initiate as much as she used to, so I have made a point of bringing some laughter into our visits. It relaxes both of us and sometimes we're surprised at how our laughter cheers those around us. It's contagious!

Consider this: One care facility resident has been an expert joke teller all his life. His family and friends keep his storehouse of jokes full. Every time they hear a new tasteful joke they write it down and remember to tell him on their next visit or phone conversation. After they have shared a good healthy laugh together, he enjoys retelling the jokes to his friends within the care facility.

Sharing the Care

My loved one complains about not being able to sleep well at night. It appears the staff makes sure he maintains a regular schedule for sleep time and awake time. The amount of exercise he gets is appropriate for his abilities. I'm trying to figure out what factors are contributing to his apparent insomnia.

Consider this: Make sure the staff limits the time your relative spends in bed during the day. Is he napping too much—even while sitting up? He might be on medications that sedate him during the day. If so, talk to his physician about changing them. Check to see if he is drinking beverages with caffeine in the evenings. If he is, suggest de-decaffeinated products. Is there a possibility your loved one is depressed? Ask him if his bed is comfortable enough to insure a good sleep.

Sharing the Care

Although this is a joyous time of the year, I'm aware that depression can be a frequent holiday visitor. I'm particularly conscious of my loved one's emotional stability. She has suffered many losses. She has been separated from people and things that are dear to her.

Consider this: Holidays and even wintertime can be depressing to some individuals. Your relative may be bogged down with memories of past holidays. If you sense she is depressed, encourage her to talk about it. Be sensitive to the amount of celebrating that is appropriate for her this year. Put thought and compassion into your special holiday time with her.

Sharing the Care

I'm a real life caregiver and I'm a real person. There are limits on my stamina. I am often caught between many responsibilities. I make mistakes. I'm not perfect. And, I'm certainly not Wonder Woman!

Consider this: Most of us overdo during the holidays. We push ourselves to please others—often beyond our limits and to our own detriment. Be careful of yourself this holiday season. Pick and chose the things you can and want to do. Decide what is important. Eliminate excess in all things. Get plenty of rest. Relax and just take pleasure in the people around you.

Sharing the Care

I'm thankful for the rules and regulations that protect my loved one. There are many people overseeing the quality of his care. As his primary advocate, I accept my responsibility to know and understand the results of inspections of the facility.

Consider this: The Department of Health makes periodic unannounced visits to care facilities to inspect and reinforce regulations. The survey results should always be available to you. Read the Statement of Deficiencies. Be particularly observant of the facility's Plan of Correction. The inspectors will return to make sure deficiencies are corrected.

Sharing the Care

I go through the doors that are opened to me. I don't stand on the outside looking in at others. I don't construct walls that separate me from those I love. I won't shield myself from sharing both laughter and tears with them.

Consider this: We sometimes try to protect ourselves with invisible walls. It might look like we're present, when we are actually just on the fringes—out of reach emotionally to those who need us and out of touch with our own needs. We must not cheat others or ourselves. We must risk emotional hurts. Only then will we be able to truly experience the fullness of life.

Sharing the Care

Joy to the world! A very simple message. A simple plan for mankind. How often we try to complicate it. God's gift is not just for today. It's for every day—and it's eternal.

Consider this: Slow down and experience the joy of the day. If the day is difficult for you, look around you. Help someone else. Reach out to others. Share hope and peace with someone else. It's a sure way to increase your own.

Sharing the Care

I've always been told it's the little things in life that matter most. I believe this is very true in the care facility situation. The small things I do for my loved one are the ones she values the highest. They seem to reach her heart more than the big things.

Consider this: Brushing someone's hair provides touch and sends a message of caring. Gently wiping a mouth or providing moisture to dry lips are acts of loving-kindness. Giving your relative a massage with pleasant smelling lotion may be most appreciated. Think of what you would want someone to do for you if you were in your relative's place.

Sharing the Care

It's amazing to me how the simple things make such big differences in our quality of life. Observances of small details make the difference between a home that is comfortable and comforting and a home that is merely tolerable.

Consider this: The use of round tables in the dining room is more conducive to conversations and comfort. Everyone is in view of others at their table. People can see and hear each other without straining their heads. Additional chairs fit in the circle with little effort. And, there are no sharp corners to harm delicate skin.

Sharing the Care

A certain amount of routine is good in everyone's life. But, too much of something could become monotonous. Boredom can set in and zap creativity.

Consider this: When television viewing is too routine, self-initiated activities decline. Even if your relative is bedridden, there are many activities and interests she can pursue. However, she may need a nudge from you or the activity director. Suggest books to read, books to listen to on audiotape, or music to listen to as an alternative to television. Large playing cards and solitaire boards can provide hours of entertainment. Some craft projects may even be appropriate.

Sharing the Care

Oddly enough, I've gotten to know my loved one better in this setting than when we were both busy going our own ways. In the past, we were always involved in separate activities. The circumstances and the surroundings of today have slowed us both down. We finally have the time to nurture the invisible bond that always existed between us.

Consider this: In this busy world, family members don't always make the time to get to know each other as real people. In fact, we take each other for granted most of the time. The slowed down pace of the care facility world forces all visitors, residents and us alike to sit down together and get acquainted.

Sharing the Care

Some things are just out of my control. In fact, when it comes right down to it—most things are. The only thing I can really control is me.

Consider this: Each person is in control of his own attitude and reactions to his life experiences. We are not responsible for anyone else's outlook on life. We each choose our own views. We can be supportive of others on their journey through life, but we can't take responsibility for someone else's attitude. Remember, no two people will perceive the same experience in the same way.

Sharing the Care

As I reflect on this care facility experience, I see many changes—changes in me and in others. I see growth in all of us. We've learned to work together. The partnership is good and it continues to improve.

Consider this: Sharing the care is a commitment to working together for quality. It's knowing what really matters. It's respect for each person's part in the care. It's recognizing everyone's dignity and value. It takes time and energy, but it's time well spent. It's letting God work through each of us. It's Love at work and Love never fails!

Index

A

ABANDONMENT: 3,231
ABILITY: 154,168
ACCEPTANCE: 6,16,152,153,176,230,280,283,
ACTIVITIES: 22,41,47,49,56,60,81,87,90,
118,125,144,149,156,164,166,171,188,219,239,
267,279,314,318,342,362
ADJUSTMENT: 3,5,49,331
AFFECTION: 225
AFFIRMATION: 245,268,283
AGING: 73,89,167,191,193,243,340
ANGER: 95,99
ANIMALS: 34,159,181,197,236
ANXIETY: 20,227,278
APPEARANCE: 27,72
APPRECIATION: 77,108,153,283
ART: 103,118,125,306
ATTENTION: 31,343
ATTITUDE: 21,34,35,37,40,85,88,137,232,236,
281,301,315, 330,341
AWARENESS: 85

B

BALANCE: 3,29,67,82,231,257,290,338,351
BATHING: 227
BEDTIME: 56,281,316

E

F

S

W

The authors,
Lyn and Bill Roche,
can be contacted by e-mail:
<u>sharingthecare@digital.net</u>

Need more copies of Sharing The Care?

To place credit card orders call 1-800-596-2455
or
Order on line at www.sharingthecarethebook.com

Checks: Make payable to Journey Publications
          3540 E. Saint Andrews Drive
          Avon Park, FL 33825-6066

Cost is: $14.95 per copy
Plus: 3.50 shipping & handling

(Add $1.75 shipping & handling each additional copy.)
Florida residents add 7% sales tax to book price.

Discounts are available on orders of five or more.
Check our web site or call for discount rates.

Also be sure to visit our web site for information
regarding other resource items and information on
Seminars!

Web site: www.sharingthecarethebook.com
Email: sharingthecare@digital.net
Toll free telephone number: 1-800-596-2455

Journey Publications . . . Caring enough to share.